How to Get
Kids To Eat Great
and Love It!

by Christine Wood, M.D.

Director of Operations: Robin L. Howland
Project Manager: Bryan K. Howland
Book and Cover Design: m2design group
Proofreader: Laurie Gibson

10 9 8 7 6 5 4 3 2 1
ISBN 1-58000-097-5

KidsEatGreat, Inc.
P.O. Box 1490
Verdi, NV 89439
www.kidseatgreat.com

Griffin Publishing Group
2908 Oregon Court, Suite I-5
Torrance, CA 90503
www.griffinpublishing.com

Manufactured in the United States of America

Disclaimer

Acknowledgments

Thanks to all in the USANA family, especially Susan Waitley, Ray Strand, M.D., Ladd McNamara, M.D., Bart Moore, M.D., Sharon Taylor, M.D., Patty Abraham, Susan Gordon, Cindy Bennett and Dr. Myron Wentz. Thanks to all the others I have met in USANA who have encouraged and appreciated my passion for healthy children.

Thanks to my associates at El Camino Pediatrics who have been supportive and have been the best group of doctors to work with in the world: Fred Frumin, M.D., Laura Nathanson, M.D., Rosalind Dockweiler, M.D., Gary Gross, M.D., Nick Levy, M.D., Sangita Bhasin, M.D., Julie Snyder-Block, M.D., Ron Park, M.D., and Melissa Reinhardt, M.D. Thanks to all the terrific staff members who make our office run efficiently and pleasantly.

Thanks to all my patients and families who have taught me so much over the years.

Thanks to Joyce Edelbrock, who encouraged and edited the first edition of this book.

Thanks to all the terrific staff at Griffin Publishing Group who supported the revision and creation of the second edition.

Dedication

To my wonderful mother, Margaret Ito, who has always been a pillar of strength.

In loving memory of her husband, my father, Rikuma Ito, I dedicate this book.

Both have been the ultimate teachers in my life.

To my husband, Kevin, and my son, Warren, whose love and laughter I treasure every day.

About the Author

Christine Wood, M.D., has been a practicing pediatrician for sixteen years and is the author of the book *How to Get Kids to Eat Great & Love It!* (KidsEatGreat, Inc., 1999) and maintains two web sites at www.callyourped.com (1996) and www.kidseatgreat.com (1998).

She lectures to physicians on the topic of nutritional medicine for children and gives seminars to parents on healthy lifestyle practices for children. She has been a guest writer for *Newsweek,* a special edition released in October 2000, called "Your Child." Her information has been cited in magazines including *Redbook* (January 2001), *Fit Pregnancy* (May 2001), *Family Life, Wasatch Parent,* and *Great Life Magazine.* She is a frequent guest on radio shows nationwide in which she informs parents about the critical need for proper nutrition for their children. An international nutritional company, USANA, has selected her to be one of four physicians on their Medical Advisory Board. She has lectured in the United States, Canada, Australia, New Zealand, and Japan.

She attended the University of Detroit and received her medical degree from the University of Michigan. She completed her pediatric residency at Children's Hospital of Los Angeles. She received her lactation educator certification from the University of California, San Diego.

Dr. Wood explains that she found a need to address the questions her patients repeatedly ask regarding the role nutrition plays in the health of their children. Dr. Wood says, "Parents need to realize what an important job they have to teach their kids healthy eating habits, to use proper nutritional supplementation, and to participate in regular physical activity. Parents must start today, model a healthy lifestyle, and do all they can to create children who will eat healthy and be active. It is perhaps the greatest gift we can give our children . . . *the gift of health now and long into their future.*"

Table of Contents

SECTION C: The War Against Diseases— Now & Long Into Adulthood

APPENDIX

Introduction

How do you get kids to eat great and love it? My experience as a mother and as a pediatrician tells me that parents make a tremendous difference and they can influence their kids in a positive way. Some seemingly difficult problems often have some very simple solutions.

Feeding kids today is a complex task. Parents can easily become overwhelmed with information overload about food choices, nutritional content, environmental issues, and feeding practices. Why is nutrition so critically important, and what is the impact on your children's future? Why has feeding kids right become so complex? This book will help you sort out that information and give you answers to many of your eating problems.

As parents, we often find ourselves busy and overwhelmed with jobs, commuting, and raising kids. Caretakers, grandparents, and daycare providers are influencing our kids more often and may have different ideas about raising them and about what they should and should not eat. Getting a healthy home-cooked meal on the table can be a challenge. As a working mother, I know this firsthand. We struggle to offer healthy food choices for our children as they clamor for fast foods, sugary cereals, the latest advertised candy, or a fat-filled snack for their lunch box.

Although we as parents understand that good nutrition is important for our children, many children eat a diet high in sugar and fat, low in calcium, and low in fruits and vegetables. How our children eat has a great deal to do with what they learn from the people around them. These messages are received in subtle and not-so-subtle ways.

Feeding children is a balancing act. There is something we might call the "Battle Zone Diet," defined as: the more you force, the less they eat. Battle zones create stress and conflict at the dinner table. But somehow, we must get the message across about healthy eating to our children. I am not talking about enforcing strict eating habits and setting rigid rules. As kids grow up, they will become more independent about their food choices and eating habits. Parents can't expect to be in control and "police" every morsel of food their children eat. So the perplexing question is, *"How do we teach kids to accept and develop healthy eating habits?"*

We can all think of a child who seems to eat all sorts of vegetables and fruits and rarely fusses about food choices, and then we can all think of a child whose main staple is macaroni and cheese. The cost to their health for continually making poor choices could be devastating. Creating healthy eating habits is a preventative health issue that needs to be taken seriously.

This book is an accumulation of my passion to help families realize the important job they have to influence the eating habits of their children in a positive way. I want to instill that passion to you, because without that passion, you will not move ahead and make the necessary changes. Unfortunately, what I find is that something devastating has to happen before we are willing to make the changes. By then, it is too late. The benefits of eating healthy and using appropriate nutritional supplementation may save a child from a degenerative disease of aging. What a wonderful gift to give to our children—health.

When I had my son, I was committed to teaching him how to eat healthy. I went back to full-time practice eight weeks after his birth and I committed to breastfeeding for a year. I bought primarily organic foods and started to do research on the environment and the environmental risks our children are experiencing. I did not want to expose him to excess processed foods and fast foods. He has profited from my efforts of developing healthy eating habits. Yes, he likes french fries and candy if they are around, but they are not around much. He loves soybeans, tofu, salad, and some days eats as many as seven or eight servings of fruits and vegetables. He often asks for fruit for dessert. He is a physically active kid who has little time to watch television. One of the benefits I found as I taught myself more about nutrition was that my husband and I were eating healthier, too. My commitment to keep my son healthy became a commitment to keep my family healthy.

The younger your child is when you start practicing healthy eating, the easier it will be later on. I have seen this reinforced over and over again by my patients. Those who choose to limit the junk and introduce a great variety of health foods throughout the early formative years seem to have an easier time keeping their kids on track with healthy eating. But whatever the age, **it is better to start *now* rather than later.** This book will give you the tools you need to start making these changes.

Discovering Nutritional Medicine

Fresh out of pediatric residency and ready to treat disease with every pharmaceutical drug imaginable, I joined a practice in Los Angeles that attracted many people interested in alternative health care. My Asian background and upbringing allowed me to be open to learning about alternative healing and I started to realize there was a place and time for non-traditional methods. Western medicine did not have all the answers.

In 1996, I had some personal improvements in allergy symptoms with the use of a nutritional supplementation program and essential fatty acids. These changes sent me down the road of research into the area of nutritional medicine—things I never learned in medical school. The research astounded me and I realized that I wanted my family to stay on a regimen of supplementation for life. I now believe using nutritional supplementation can help maintain health in a world that has created many threats to our health. This book will help you understand why clinical nutritional science is very important in maintaining health.

Topics in This Book

Topics addressed in this book include:

- How to minimize health risks found in our environment. Learn about the environmental risks our children face from pesticides, nitrates in foods, mercury in fish, water contamination, and persistent toxic chemicals.

- How to develop healthy eating habits for various age groups. Learn techniques and adjust your expectations for each age group. Learn how to handle picky eaters and how to support the overweight child.

- How to use nutritional supplementation to improve health problems. Learn nutritional principles that can help children with allergies, asthma, attention deficit disorder, and immunity challenges. Learn how a start with healthy nutrition may help avoid adult diseases such as cancer and heart disease.

What You Need to Do

Have a heart-to-heart talk with yourself, your spouse, and anyone else involved in feeding your child. Realize that what you are about to learn in this book may change the odds of diseases well into your own future and well into the future of your child. Look at yourself first. Then look at your children. Remember that day when your child was born and how innocent and wholesome he appeared. As a parent, we carry hope and love in our hearts as we acquaint ourselves with our baby. Hope . . . that we may be a good parent and offer him every opportunity to become a wonderful human being. Hope . . . that we can protect him from harm and danger. Hope . . . that he will be healthy and stay healthy. We can achieve these goals by reading about parenting or taking classes about child-rearing; by safety-proofing our home and learning CPR; by modeling and teaching a lifestyle of healthy eating habits and exercise; and by understanding environmental risks and how to use nutritional supplements as protection.

Let's do all we can to maintain the hope and love we have for our children. Their bodies will love us for it. So, let's learn **how to get kids to eat great and love it!**

Visit the Kids Eat Great web site and sign up for a
FREE nutrition newsletter at
www.kidseatgreat.com.

SECTION
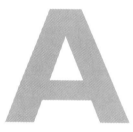
A

Our Children's World: Positive Actions to Protect Them

Chapter One
Healthy Eating for A Lifetime of Healthy Living

What parent wouldn't want to give the gift of good health and a lifetime of good eating habits to his or her children? As a parent and a pediatrician I feel very strongly that we, as parents, have a job to do in protecting and nurturing our kids. We suffer as much as our child does with every cold, fever, cut, bruise, ache, and pain. We do our best to protect them by using car seats and bike helmets, and by being watchful parents.

We would not knowingly expose our child to a deadly virus or bacteria. Yet, many parents allow unhealthy eating habits for their children, putting them at risk for disease. This is the disease that we don't see, disease that lurks under the surface, within the cells, within the arterial walls, and within the bones of our children. This is not as obvious to us, nor will it become obvious until many years down the line, perhaps, long after we're gone.

We are talking about the degenerative diseases of aging, like heart disease, stroke, arthritis, macular degeneration, diabetes, and cancer. These processes are heavily influenced by our diet, but most of the research so far has focused on the adult diet. However, many of the changes have already started in childhood. Our children must begin early and learn a healthy style of eating to give them every advantage later in life. We may be able to change their odds by understanding nutrition and nutritional supplementation and its role in preventative medicine.

Health is one of our greatest concerns of today. Many baby boomers are previewing death as they watch their parents suffer through many of the degenerative diseases of aging. We want to change our odds. Some of us are driven to pursue health by hiring fitness trainers, starting weight loss programs, trying to eat healthfully, and trying more "natural remedies" to treat disease. Emotionally, physically, and spiritually, we are seeking answers about health.

Our children need good role models when it comes to leading a healthy lifestyle. Don't think for a minute that you can't make a difference. You can. Yes, our children are influenced by advertising and marketing of unhealthy foods and by the foods at their best friend's house, but their families also influence them. When it comes to feeding our children, I see many parents allowing their children to eat piles of unhealthy food that may ultimately cause obesity, high cholesterol, heart attacks, or diabetes later in life. Why are we so careless when it comes to what our children eat?

A study from the medical journal *Pediatrics* surveyed 3,307 children, 2 to 19 years of age in the United States. Only 1 percent, that is 33 children, met all recommendations for the Food Guide Pyramid. Total intakes of fat and added sugars were well above recommended levels. The most common food intake pattern was those children not meeting any recommendations for food groups. Most children did not meet the requirements for the Recommended Daily Allowance (RDA) for vitamin B-6, calcium, iron, zinc, and fiber.[1] Our children are growing up in a fast food world, and advertisers are targeting their marketing dollars on unhealthy food choices. The truth is that most children are not getting the nutrition they need.

Our War Against Changing Health Trends

Health trends have changed drastically over the last several decades, and these trends will affect many of our children as they age. Many of these health trends, as you will learn, can be directly related to poor eating habits in our children. Nutrition impacts many aspects of health and disease. Unfortunately, poor eating habits are the norm and not the exception. Early eating patterns can set the stage for your child's growth, strength, immunity, and intelligence. It can also influence the development of diseases such as allergies, asthma, heart disease, cancer, diabetes, and osteoporosis. Many of these degenerative diseases of aging that we associate only with "old age" are occurring in younger and younger age groups and are clearly processes that start in childhood. Health trends that are influenced by nutrition include:

- **Obesity on the Rise.** Obesity now affects 1 in 5 children in the United States.[2] Obesity is the most prevalent nutritional disease of children and adolescents. From 1963 to 1980, obesity among U.S. children has increased by 54 percent in 6 to 11 year olds and by 40 percent in adolescents.[3] These obese children will most likely become obese adults and carry all the extra risks for diseases such as heart attacks, strokes, high blood pressure, and diabetes. Obesity is much easier to prevent than to cure and prevention in childhood should be our primary target.

- **Cardiovascular Disease is the Number One Killer.** Heart disease is the leading cause of death in the United States and in many Westernized countries around the world. As more countries adopt Western diets and lifestyles, the incidence of heart disease is climbing. It is estimated that healthy lifestyles—including a low-fat, high-fiber diet and exercise—can reduce the risk of heart disease by as much as 80 percent.

- **Cancer on the Rise in Children.** Federal health experts have concerns about why cancer rates are on the rise in children. Childhood cancer has risen almost 11 percent in the past decade.[4] Cancer has become the leading cause of death due to disease among children. It is second to trauma as a cause of death. In recent years, deaths from cancer have declined because of earlier detection and improved treatment, but experts are concerned that survival rates could be eclipsed because of the rising rates of new cases. Dr. Kenneth Cooper, author of the *Antioxidant Revolution,* feels that environmental toxins are in part responsible for this increase. Some experts estimate that as many as 80 percent of cancers are caused by environmental factors. Antioxidants found in foods are critical to battling the environmental effects that may lead to cancer formation. In addition, obesity can also increase the risk of developing certain types of cancer.

- **Allergies and Asthma Now Affect Millions of Children.** The 1996 statistics from the Centers for Disease Control show that asthma affects over 14 million Americans. This is nearly double the rate from 1980. Almost 5 million of these asthmatics are children. The role of air pollution and other toxins has been implicated in contributing to this rise in allergies and asthma. The diet of a developing infant and child can influence the severity and onset of allergies. Early food exposures can program a child's immune system to activate future allergies to foods and other airborne allergens, like dust, mold, and pollens.

- **Calcium Deficiency Leads to Osteoporosis.** Osteoporosis affects 25 million Americans a year and contributes to approximately 1.3 million bone fractures per year, according to the American Academy of Orthopedic Surgeons. The process of gradual bone loss occurs throughout adulthood, so what is built up early in life is critical to minimizing the effects of bone loss later in life. The average calcium intake in adolescents is about half of the RDA.[5] Our children and teens need to understand that this time in their life is their only chance at building bone.

- **Attention Deficit Disorder (ADD) and Learning Disabilities Increasing.** In the United States, ADD appears to be rising. Statistics from 1998 estimate that 3 to 5 percent of school-aged children have ADD. The influence of diet on this problem is still unclear. However, we do understand that nutrient deficiencies can affect neurologic function and may influence learning and behavior. Iron deficiency anemia can have a permanent impact on IQ potential and motor development. Fats are another very important nutrient that affect brain development, especially in infants. Breast milk is 50 percent fat and has the right type of fats that allow for optimal brain development. This will be covered in more detail in Chapter 15.

Obesity in Children: A Rapidly Growing Epidemic

A worldwide epidemic of childhood obesity is occurring. Depending on how "overweight" is defined in children, at least 11 percent and possibly as many as 25 percent of children in the United States are overweight.[6] (See p.147, "Defining 'Overweight' and 'Obese'.") The prevalence of obesity in children and adults in the United States has increased by more than 30 percent over the past decade.[7] The 1999 National Center for Health Statistics revealed that 61 percent of U.S. adults are either overweight or obese; this is 5 percent higher than estimates from 1988-1994.

There is a growing concern among health professionals about the impact of obesity in childhood and the health of future generations. We know that as children approach late childhood and adolescence, it becomes more difficult to change eating habits and shed unwanted pounds. That is why it is important to create healthy eating habits early in life.

Trends are occurring that affect the eating habits of our children, including:

- High-calorie, high-fat, ready-made foods are easily available and desired by children and adults. A hundred years ago, when fresh, locally grown foods were all that were available, people had limited food choices. Since the entry of the first TV dinners in 1954, processed foods have become more and more popular. Now with an overwhelming number of items available, it is easy to snack on crackers, chips, or cookies instead of fresh foods. There are over 12,000 new processed food choices introduced each year in the United States. Our society appears to be going through a palate change that desires these processed foods. Unfortunately, these choices are usually low in nutritional value and high in caloric density.

- Despite all the knowledge of the health benefits of regular exercise, our children are not necessarily receiving those benefits. Only about 36 percent of children participate in physical activity in school on a daily basis. Of students in grades nine through twelve, only half reported being enrolled in physical education classes.[8] Lean school budgets have forced minimal physical education requirements.

- Since the introduction of cable TV, VCR's, remote controls, Game Boy, Nintendo, and home personal computers, more sedentary options are available than ever. Researchers have found a strong correlation between the time spent watching television and being overweight.[9] According to Nielsen Media Research, children between 2 and 5 years of age watch nearly 28 hours of television a week. The average 6- to 11-year-old watches almost 24 hours of television a week. This does not even include the time spent in front of the computer or playing video games. The average adult American watches 3 hours and 43 minutes of television each day, according to a Nielsen Media Research study. This adds up to 56 days of nonstop TV per year!

- Food companies are taking advantage of all the time spent in front of the television and are marketing to our children. Watch any children's program and you will see a string of commercials for fast food restaurants, sugar-loaded cereals, candy, and soft drinks. In addition, many schools allow fast food restaurants like Pizza Hut and Taco Bell to provide the school lunch. Banks of vending machines with junk food and sodas are commonly found in middle schools and high schools. What type of message does this send to our children?

- More working parents mean that many children are home alone after school. It also means that there is less time cooking at home and more meals eaten away from home. Money spent on eating out has increased from 29 cents of every food dollar spent on snacks and meals away from home in 1970 to 40 cents in 1992.

- Individuals from a low income level may experience what has been called "food insecurity," meaning that there are periodic shortages of food. There is a high rate of being overweight among this population. The paradox of having limited food resources and being overweight is likely related to poor food choices and binge eating when food sources are available.[10]

- Concerns with violence in our society have allowed our children to become more sedentary, especially among the urban areas of the country. Children must come home and stay indoors after school because of fear of violence outside the home.

Although parents may not want to face the facts about unhealthy eating and their child's weight problems, there are health risks. **What impact does obesity have on our children?**

- It has been estimated that a poor diet and lack of activity contribute to about 300,000 preventable deaths in the United States per year, or about 1,000 deaths per day. This is second only to smoking-related deaths.[11]

- Overweight children have a higher rate of developing asthma. The rate of new asthmatics was more than double in children in the highest 20 percent of the body mass index.[12]

- Obese children have a higher risk of developing cardiovascular diseases like heart attacks, strokes, and high blood pressure as they age. Excess body fat raises cholesterol and triglyceride levels.

- Being overweight accelerates the aging process and reduces longevity. A study from Harvard researchers in 1995 showed that among a group of female nurses, modestly overweight women were 60 percent more likely to die than the thinnest women.[13] What is even more frightening is that research shows that people who were overweight as kids—regardless of their adult weight—were more likely to die earlier.[14]

- There is a rising incidence of overweight children and adolescents being diagnosed with adult-onset diabetes (type II diabetes). This type of obesity is more clearly related to being overweight. Excess fat leads to reduced efficiency of insulin, the pancreas produces more insulin and wears out, and type II diabetes is then evident. In 1970 type II diabetes made up 2 percent of new cases of diabetes in children 9 to 19 years; in 2000 this number rose to 30 to 50 percent of new cases in children.

- The increased weight bearing adds more stress to hips and knees and overweight children can develop an orthopedic condition called *slipped femoral epiphysis*, where the head of the thigh bone, called the femur, slips out of the hip joint. Also, arthritis is more common in overweight people.

- The World Health Organization (WHO) estimates that 1 in 4 kidney and gallbladder cancer cases, 1 in 10 colon, and 1 in 12 breast cancers in postmenopausal women are related to obesity. Health experts estimate that healthier diets and exercise could reduce cancer cases by 30 to 40 percent—that would be 3 to 4 million cases—worldwide every year.

- Obese children face significant negative psychosocial consequences such as discrimination from their peers and low self-esteem. The obsession with being thin can lead to other eating problems, such as anorexia and bulimia.

National Report Card:
We're Failing Our Children Nutritionally

In 1998, the American Medical Association released a Children's Nutrition Study that surveyed over 700 American parents. The findings include:

- Nearly all parents (99 percent) agreed, "it is important for my child to eat nutritious foods." The majority (91 percent) said that it's important to restrict the amount of sugars consumed, and 84 percent believed dietary fat reduction was important.

- Soft drinks were picked by more parents (27 percent) as their child's "preferred" drink over any other beverage.

- Children ate fatty foods (like chips and other snacks) nearly five times per week on average.

- Despite the above statistics, three out of four parents said they were "not that concerned" that their child "drinks too many soft drinks" or "only likes junk food."

- Eighty percent of parents say they are familiar with the Food Guide Pyramid. However, less than half said they used it to plan their children's meals.

Other studies have found such trends as:

- Teenagers in the United States now drink twice as much soda as milk. The average soda consumption in males between ages 13 and 18 is 3 or more cans of soda per day and 10 percent drink 7 or more cans a day. For 13 to 18-year-old girls, the average intake is more than 2 cans a day and 10 percent drink more than 5 cans a day.[15]

- Of 168 U.S. preschoolers followed in a week-long nutrition study, none ate the recommended five daily servings of fruits and vegetables. Most ate less than a half serving of vegetables and two servings of fruit per day. About half of the fruit servings were in the form of juice.[16]

- Only one in five children consumed five or more serving of fruits and vegetables a day. Nearly one-quarter of all vegetables consumed by children and adolescents were french fries.[17]

- Breakfast cereal has become a major source of children's nutrients, despite the fact that we know they should be receiving their nutrients from a variety of foods. Cereal has become the main source of iron and vitamin A for children and the second largest source of vitamin C. Fruit juices make up about 14 percent of total vitamin C intake.[18]

We are obviously not doing a good job when it comes to feeding our children. Things have to change if we are going to make a difference in their future health.

Free Radicals:
Aging Our Children and Causing Degenerative Diseases

Our children are aging before our very eyes. We marvel at how they are growing, developing, and learning new skills at a fast pace. Aunt Jenny who hasn't seen her niece for a long time will certainly comment, "My, how she's grown!" The growth of our children is a way of measuring time. However, aging occurs under the surface of missing teeth and bigger shoes and clothes.

Aging is occurring at the cellular level in our children. In order to understand this, we need to comprehend the free radical theory of aging and oxidative stress. Free radicals are unstable oxygen molecules with a single electron that are constantly being formed and bombarding our bodies. It is a result of our normal metabolism as our cells burn fuel for energy. Free radicals increase as a result of exposure to air and water pollution, stress, excess exercise, environmental toxins, smoke, radiation, fatty foods, and sun exposure. Free radicals may lead to cellular, tissue, and DNA damage and increase the risk of more than fifty degenerative diseases of aging. These diseases include cancer, heart disease, stroke, arthritis, cataracts, and macular degeneration.

Free radical damage starts early in life and is cumulative. Cancer development is due to DNA damage brought about by years of free radical damage. Most cancers probably develop over 10 to 20 years and are diagnosed in their last stages.

Our children are experiencing the effects of degenerative diseases earlier than we think. Autopsies of young Americans showed that fatty streaks, which are the first signs of atherosclerosis, were noted in the hearts of the majority of children 10 to 14 years of age. Over 5 percent had more advanced lesions.[19]

Imagine if you could look into the arteries of your child and see the progression of this disease. Would you change your family's eating habits? Today's child may be tomorrow's cardiac patient. Programs aimed at preventing heart disease "must begin in childhood or adolescence," according to a report published in *The Journal of the American Medical Association*. This statement was based on a report of Americans between the ages of 15 and 34 that showed some people had more advanced raised lesions in the heart arteries at these ages. Dr. Jack P. Strong of Louisiana State University Medical Center, one of the researchers, stated, "It's going to take more than just the doctors—it's the parents, it's the schools, it's the students and young people themselves knowing that they need to start early—that's the main message."[20]

Antioxidants in Nutritional Foods and Supplements: Fighting Free Radicals

Antioxidants are an important way to defend against free radical damage. Antioxidants readily give up an electron to stabilize the free radicals and render them harmless. Our bodies produce a variety of antioxidants, but they need outside sources from food and a supplement program. The most powerful antioxidants are vitamin C, vitamin E, and the precursor to vitamin A, beta-carotene. Other antioxidants that are now recognized as important include coenzyme Q10 and bioflavonoids. A host of supporting minerals is also necessary to optimize free radical neutralization.

The best place to get these antioxidants is through fruits and vegetables. Research shows there is a protective effect of fruits and vegetables against a variety of diseases. In men 45 to 65 years of age, who were followed for more than 20 years, it was determined that for every increase of 3 servings of fruits or vegetables a day, there was a 22 percent decrease in the risk of stroke.[21] Dr. Bruce Ames, a well-known cancer researcher, found that people with the lowest dietary intake of fruits and vegetables have twice the cancer rate.[22]

Our first goal should be to have our children eat a variety of fruits and vegetables. Our second goal should be to understand the role that sensible nutritional supplementation has in defending against free radical damage. Chapter 3 will address this issue.

Chapter One
roundup
Healthy Eating for a Lifetime of Healthy Living

- Be aware of the changing trends of today:

    children are eating less healthy foods,

    children are less physically active, and

    children are exposed to dangerous environmental toxins.

- Children are becoming more vulnerable to:

    free radical damage,

    degenerative diseases, and

    obesity.

- Parents need to model:

    good eating habits and

    an active lifestyle for better health.

- Parents need to:

    fight against the giant money interests of highly advertised, nutritionally deprived foods and

    guide their children to making healthy food choices.

- Parents today need to understand the role that nutritious food and supplementation has in:

    neutralizing free radical damage,

    improving immunity and health, and

    reducing the risks of degenerative diseases.

- When parents do this, they are giving the gift of health to their children.

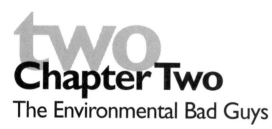

Chapter Two

The Environmental Bad Guys

Who are the Environmental Bad Guys?

Should we blame certain health problems on the environment and complain about how bad things have gotten?

Or should we become informed about what's happening in our world and do something about protecting our children and ourselves?

The information in this chapter may leave you with more questions than answers. I realize that some of this information may seem overwhelming and frightening. Rather than feeling frightened, feel empowered so that you can make some simple changes to protect your family.

Consumers are more aware today of food, water, and environmental safety issues. The media has reported outbreaks of Giardia (a parasite) in our water supply, E.coli (a bacterium) in our meats, and hepatitis A (a virus) in strawberries from Mexico. A study from the Hartman Group found that 53 percent of consumers are concerned about pesticide residues in food, and 55 percent believe manmade hormones and antibiotics do not belong in meat. Seventy percent think organic products are better for one's health. Roughly 33 percent of Americans are buying organic food at least once or twice a month. We assume that our foods are safe and nutritious, but let's look at who decides what is safe as well as what is happening within our food supply.

How Are Safety Standards for Pesticides Met?

Toxicology is far from an exact science when it comes to estimating the safety standards of pesticides. Current pesticide standards, called *tolerances*, are based on the assumption that people are exposed to only one pesticide at a time. Studies to evaluate safety standards are done with animals because it is unethical to test toxic safety standards in humans. An additional "uncertainty factor" is then added as a theoretical safety margin for humans. Is it reliable to assume that a chemical is safe in humans because it is safe in an animal? The chemical DDT (dichlorodiphenyltricholorethane) was widely used until studies linked it to cancer development. However, we are still paying the price with DDT due to its inability to be easily degraded and its continued presence in our food supply. Humans are exposed to other factors like multiple toxins, air and water pollution, pharmaceutical drugs, malnourishment, and disease that may interact and make a person more vulnerable to side effects. There are clearly limitations of animal testing of pesticides.

What Is the Government Doing for Our Children?

Safety standards are based on the adult male, and they presently do not consider the vulnerability of children. A landmark report from the National Academy of Sciences in 1993 entitled "Pesticides in the Diets of Infants and Children" recognized that infants and children are at the highest risk from toxic substances, but often they are the least protected. This report encouraged the federal government to change its scientific and regulatory procedures to protect children. Here are several factors from this report that need to be recognized:

- Children have fast metabolisms, less varied diets, and are particularly vulnerable to the effects of pesticides.

- Their ability to activate, detoxify, and excrete toxins is different than adults and generally they are less able to handle toxic chemicals.

- Because of their smaller size, children are exposed to higher levels of pesticides per unit of body weight.

- Measurements of pesticide residues tend to focus on foods eaten by the average adult; children's diets are underrepresented.

- Effects of multiple exposures to pesticides may be greater than the sum of effects from separate exposures and must be evaluated.

- Better tests and more data are needed to evaluate concerns about the effects of toxins in children.

- Safety standards should apply to multiple health effects, not just cancer, including harm to the nervous, immune, endocrine, and reproductive systems.

- The effects of non-dietary sources of pesticide exposure combined with dietary sources of exposure need to be evaluated.

The Food Quality Protection Act, passed unanimously by Congress in 1996, requires that all pesticides be safe for infants and children and promises to reassess the levels of pesticide residues allowed in food. The law also stipulates that combined exposures to pesticides be considered when setting safety standards. The United States Environmental Protection Agency (EPA) is committed to increasing protection for infants and children, but new standards may take years to develop. The agency has until 2006 to ensure that all old pesticides meet new standards. Many environmental groups have been critical of the EPA missing deadlines set by Congress to review nearly 10,000 pesticides and set safety standards to protect infants and young children. Consumers Union, an advocacy group and publisher of *Consumer Reports* magazine, published an analysis in February 2001 titled "A Report Card for the EPA: Successes and Failures in Implementing the Food Quality Protection Act." They gave the EPA a "D" for its efforts in reducing dietary risks, citing slow and incomplete progress in this area.

The Reality of Pesticides

Consumer Reports has published two recent reports on pesticides in foods: one in January 1998 and one in March 1999. The main concern raised in these articles is how pesticides affect our children and the vulnerability of children to current standards. Consumers Union has criticized the EPA for not providing basic information about pesticides for consumers. Highlights from these articles include:

- The pesticide levels on nearly all produce were within legal limits but may not be at levels safe for children.

- Domestic produce had more pesticides than imported produce in two-thirds of the cases.

- Of twenty-seven foods tested between 1994 and 1997, seven—**apples, grapes, green beans, peaches, pears, spinach, and winter squash**—had the highest toxicity score. A high toxicity score does not necessarily mean a person is at high risk when eating these foods; it depends on how often and how much of the item a person eats relative to that person's body weight.

- A single sample of spinach had up to 14 different pesticides. One in 13 spinach samples had pesticide residues that exceeded the safe daily limit in a single serving for a 44-pound child.

- Foods with a very low toxicity score included apple juice, bananas, broccoli, canned peaches, milk, orange juice, and canned or frozen peas and corn.

Consumer Reports concluded that "parents might want to be careful about the types and amounts of fruits and vegetables they serve their children—while still making sure they get plenty of healthful produce. While peeling can greatly reduce pesticide residues on many fruits and vegetables, it can't eliminate them."

Organic produce may contain pesticides and other chemicals, but generally have been found to have fewer residues compared to conventional produce. Although the information about pesticides is unsettling to any parent, we must accept that we have exposures to toxins, and take measures to reduce some of the risks. (See the last section of this chapter.)

The most important point is that we must continue serving lots of fruits and vegetables. These are very necessary for a healthy diet. Don't let being an informed consumer scare you away from antioxidants in fruits and vegetables that may be your child's best protection against cancer, heart disease, and other degenerative diseases. The American Academy of Pediatrics states, "Despite the theoretical risk of pesticide residues . . . a diet rich in fruits and vegetables is the most healthful diet that children can consume."

Facts On Pesticides

- The primary concern with pesticides is the possibility of acute poisoning. The long-term effects are now felt to be equally as important. Farmers who work with pesticides seem to have a higher risk of cancer than nonfarmers. Pesticides may not only increase the risk of cancer, but can affect the nervous, endocrine, immune, and reproductive systems. Infants, unborn children, and young children are especially at risk.

- Resistance to pesticides is on the rise. It takes two to five applications of pesticides today to achieve the same effects as one application in the early 1970's.

- Pesticides are found in drinking water supplies in farm states. A study of 5,000 water samples in wells and rivers on farms have shown that half the wells and nearly all the streams contain at least one pesticide.

These facts were accumulated from Consumers Union.[23]

Persistent Toxic Chemicals

One class of toxic chemicals, *persistent organic pollutants* (POPs), is of particular concern. This group of toxins includes industrial chemicals and pesticides. These are chemicals that do not disintegrate easily in our environment and travel long distances globally by air and by water. The United Nations Environment Programme sponsored an international agreement that recognizes that a worldwide effort to stop contamination of our food supply must occur in a cooperative fashion to make an impact.

What is most disturbing is that these toxic chemicals are present in our everyday foods despite the fact that they have been banned for years in the United States. They build up in body fat and concentrate to higher levels as they make their way up the food chain. The two most prevalent POPs in our food supply are dieldrin and DDE. Dieldrin is a toxic organochlorine pesticide and DDE is a breakdown product of DDT, both banned since the 1970's. Dioxins and furans are by-products of the manufacturing and burning of plastics that contain chlorine and continue to be released globally. Dioxins and polychlorinated biphenyls (PCBs) are found in the highest concentration in fatty meats and dairy products. High-fat processed foods will also contain higher levels of these chemicals. These chemicals are associated with cancer, immune system suppression, nervous system disorders, and disruption of the reproductive and hormonal systems. Health problems such as cancer, learning disorders, poor immune function, reproductive issues (such as low sperm count and endometriosis) have been linked to exposure to POPs.

Many chemicals that have been banned in the United States still find their way into our food supply because they are still produced and stored in other countries. An analysis from the Pesticide Action Network North America's report titled "Nowhere to Hide" found that a hypothetical daily meal plan for four U.S. regions would deliver between 63 and 70 exposures to POPs per day.[24]

Top 10 Foods Most Contaminated
with Persistent Toxic Chemicals

From "Nowhere to Hide, Persistent Toxic Chemicals in the U.S. Food Supply," report from the Pesticide Action Network North America; March 2001.

Butter	Popcorn
Cantaloupe	Radishes
Cucumber/pickles	Spinach
Meatloaf	Summer squash
Peanuts	Winter squash

The Link Between Toxic Chemicals and Health

Health experts are concerned about the role environmental toxins play in childhood disease. The EPA notes the lack of awareness by the medical community of the environmental health threats to children. In April 1998 the EPA released the report, "Pesticides and National Strategies for Health Care Providers." It stated that 43 percent of chemicals have no basic toxicity data, and full basic data exists for only 7 percent of chemicals. It stated that this lack of information " . . . is always surprising to physicians, who are used to dealing with pharmaceuticals, where we have a lot of information."

The Environmental Working Group, a research organization that advocates lower exposure to pesticides, examined federal data on 4,000 children's eating habits and compared them to government test results for residue of a popular class of pesticides on 80,000 samples of food from 1992 to 1995. They estimated that 1.1 million children every day eat food that, even after it is washed or processed, contains an unsafe dose of 13 organophosphate insecticides. Just over 100,000 of those children exceeded the EPA safe daily dosage level for adults by 10 times or more. Organophosphates have been used for more than 40 years, and two-thirds of the insecticide treatments in the United States involve organophosphates.[25]

Organophosphates have been implicated in causing nervous system damage. Exposure to organophosphates in children occurs when their brains and nervous systems are most vulnerable. The EPA is presently considering banning or restricting this group of pesticides. The agency has already lowered the safe daily limit for 19 of some 40 organophosphates.

Additional research shows a link between environmental toxins and health problems in children, including:

- A study reported in the *American Journal of Public Health*, February 1995, stated, "use of home pesticides may be associated with some types of childhood cancer."[26]

- Frequent occupational exposure to pesticides or home pesticides was most strongly associated with childhood leukemia and brain cancer. This association was greater than either professional extermination or the use of garden pesticides.[27]

- Particularly vulnerable are developing fetuses. Exposure to POPs at this critical time may manifest as health problems years later or even in their offspring. PCBs are present in high concentrations in the Hudson River around New York. The New York State Department of Health advises pregnant women not to consume fish from these waters. PCBs affect the neurodevelopment of children. Those who were exposed prenatally were observed to have low birth weight, delayed developmental milestones, and lower IQs than unexposed siblings.[28] In addition, women who ate Lake Ontario fish for three or more years took longer to get pregnant compared to women who ate no fish from the lake.[29]

Genetically Engineered Foods

More media coverage about genetically engineered (GE) food is getting the attention of consumers around the world. GE crops are plants with insertions of one or more new genes in the DNA. The difference between GE and past traditional cross-breeding is that cross-breeding was only able to occur between similar species. With GE, any gene from a plant, animal, bacterium, fungus, or virus can be inserted into the DNA of other organism. The concern is that these new genetic transformations may create unforeseen health effects that may be difficult to test for or predict. About one-fourth of U.S. cropland is planted with GE crops, making the United States the world's largest producer. In 1999, about 50 percent of U.S. soybeans, 33 percent of corn, and 55 percent of cotton were GE varieties. Concerns about GE foods include:

- Allergens. New proteins appearing in foods may cross-react and set up allergic reactions. The genetically engineered corn called *StarLink* was removed from human consumption because of concerns about potential allergic reactions.

- Toxins. Bovine growth hormone used in milk production may have adverse health effects. (See next section.)

- Reduced nutritional quality. Some GE foods may have less nutritional quality. A study found that the phytoestrogen compounds in GE soybeans were lower than in non-GE soybeans. These are the compounds that have been found to be protective against heart disease and cancer.

One of the major issues consumers face is that GE products are not labeled as such in the United States. Many other countries, such as Europe, Japan, South Korea, Thailand, and New Zealand, have GE regulations and labeling requirements.

Hormones and Antibiotics in Meat

The European Union (EU) banned the use of synthetic hormones in meat and meat products in 1988. The EU is presently carrying out an additional risk assessment of the safety of hormones in meat and its effect on humans. The FDA in the United States continues to reassure consumers that hormones are safe in meats because of the tiny amount that is used in animals. Only a small fraction is transmitted to the humans who consume meat. These hormones, anabolic steroids, are used in the United States and other countries (e.g. Australia and Canada) to make cattle larger and leaner. In April 1999 the EU banned beef imports from the United States. The EU's commission stated, "This action has been taken to protect consumer health in the EU."

In addition, dairy cattle are injected with a genetically engineered growth hormone, called bovine somatotropin (BST) or recombinant bovine growth hormone (rBGH), to increase the production of milk by the cow. In a March 1999 press release the chairman of The Cancer Prevention Coalition, Dr. Samuel S. Epstein, shared concerns about rBGH and called on the FDA to immediately ban milk from cows injected with this hormone. Scientific studies from the EU have shown elevated levels of insulin-like growth factor-1 (IGF-1) in milk from these cows. Epidemiological studies indicate a link between excess levels of IGF-1 and breast and prostate cancer. Dr. Epstein also shared concerns about the antibiotic use that is necessary in these cows because of the high rate of mastitis (breast infections) in these cows.

The use of these antibiotics in our meats is a concern. Some 60 to 80 percent of all cattle, sheep, and poultry in the United States will receive antibiotics at some point. Researchers are trying to determine if and how much of a role this widespread antibiotic use may have in creating antibiotic resistance of bacteria in humans. A report from the National Academy of Sciences stated, "Bacteria that resist antibiotics can be passed from food animals to humans, but not enough is known to determine the public health risks posed by such transmission."[30]

Studies have shown that people who eat more red meat are at more risk of developing certain types of cancer. The Nurses Health Study, which enrolled over 80,000 nurses, found that the risk of colon cancer was almost double for those women who ate the most animal fat over those who ate the least.[31] Prostate cancer has also been linked to increased intake of animal fat, particularly red meat. Research trying to link breast cancer and a high-fat diet has met with mixed results. The National Research Council's Committee on Diet and Health reviewed all studies linking fat intake and breast cancer. They concluded "fat intake early in life may have a greater influence on breast cancer risk than intake later in life."

As consumers, we need to make our choices, but concerns are increasing about the safety of meat and meat products. We know that vegetarians are generally healthier and have lower risks of heart disease and cancer. Eating a low-fat, low red meat diet will not guarantee immunity to heart disease and cancer later in life. But since we know that there are some risks with a heavy meat diet, how much risk do we take? This is a decision every family and person must make, but it seems that moderation is important when it comes to red meat.

Mercury

Mercury contamination is another environmental issue that may be putting our children at risk. Mercury is found naturally in the environment; it is released into our atmosphere by degassing from the Earth's crust and oceans. It has also been placed there through industrial pollution. It dissolves in water and is converted to a more toxic form called *methyl mercury*. Fish and shellfish accumulate this metal. The bigger and more predatory the fish, the more likely it will have contamination. Shark, swordfish, and large tuna are most frequently contaminated at higher levels. Fresh-water fish can also have mercury contamination.

Historically, serious mercury intoxication has occurred in humans. In Minimata, Japan, 111 people died or became very ill from eating fish contaminated for an extended period of time with mercury from industrial waste. Neurological problems such as numbness and tingling, stumbling gait, difficulty in speech, tunnel vision and impaired hearing, tremors, and jerking motions were noted. In a report by Sallie Bernard, "Autism: a Novel Form of Mercury Poisoning," she compares characteristics of autistic spectrum disorder to the movement and sensory dysfunction found in mercury poisoning.[32] There are some eerie similarities. Although this is not the whole answer to autism, mercury's role in certain cases of autism needs to be investigated and clarified.

The population considered most at risk for serious effects from mercury is pregnant women and infants. The effects may pose serious permanent consequences to the developing brain. In March 2001 the Food and Drug Administration (FDA) released a consumer advisory on the risks of mercury in fish, which stated:

- Pregnant women and women of childbearing age who might become pregnant should not eat shark, king mackerel, swordfish, or tilefish because of their high mercury content.
- It is prudent for children and nursing mothers not to eat these fish as well.
- Children and pregnant women may eat up to 12 ounces per week of other varieties of cooked fish.

State fish advisories vary in their statements about fish. Some states have adopted a zero-risk approach and advise consumers not to eat certain species.

Facts About Fish

Nutritional Value: Fish is a nutrient-dense protein and some fish (the fatty types) are high in the important omega-3 fats. (See p. 55, "Fats: The Good, the Bad, and the Ugly.") It is a good source of vitamin B-12 and many are rich in iron. Fatty fish have many of the heart-healthy fats and brain-healthy fats and is a good food choice for kids. Fish highest in omega-3 fats are salmon, albacore and bluefin tuna steaks, sardines, rainbow trout, and mackerel.

Contamination: Concerns about toxins (like mercury and PCBs) are most critical for the developing brain of the fetus (during pregnancy) and young infants.

Farmed fish vs. wild fish: Farmed fish are fed a different diet than wild fish. Farmed fish were found to have lower omega-3 fats, but because there is more control over their environment, there may be less contaminants.

Fried fish and fish sticks: When fish is fried, the addition of the omega-6 fats and trans fats decreases the benefits of the omega-3 fats found in the fish. It is the least nutritious way to eat fish. Fish sticks are usually made from lean fish that have only small amounts of omega-3 fats. Make your own healthier fish sticks by breading salmon or tuna in strips with eggs and whole grain flour and baking them.

Canned tuna fish: *Consumer Reports* (June 2001) discussed the FDA recommendations because the FDA did not mention canned tuna as being a species to avoid for vulnerable individuals. An EPA report suggested that the FDA recommendations may be inadequate. The actual level of mercury exposure that the EPA considers safe is one-fourth the level that the FDA uses as its standard (1 part per million is the current FDA standard). Guidelines must be based on how much an individual eats and the individual's body weight. Light tuna tends to have less mercury than white (albacore) tuna. What Consumers Union figured is that a 132-pound woman could consume up to 9 ounces of light tuna or 5 ounces of white tuna a week (this assumes that no other sources of mercury ingestion occur) or a 44-pound child could eat 3 ounces of light tuna or 1.5 ounces of white tuna a week (about 1 tuna fish sandwich a week). *Consumer Reports* suggest limiting fish with higher mercury levels until age 5 and possibly for a few years more. My recommendations for children would be to limit children under 45 pounds to no more than one tuna sandwich a month.

Nitrates

Hot dogs and bologna are typical "kid foods," but they contain risks if eaten in large amounts. Nitrates are preservatives found in virtually all cooked and cured meats, like luncheon meats, bacon, sausages, ham, and hot dogs. Nitrates have a cosmetic function in that they preserve the pinkish color of meats. When nitrates combine with gastric juices in the stomach, they form a chemical called *nitrosamine*. Nitrosamines have been found to be carcinogenic in most species of animals tested. A study from the University of Southern California in 1994 found higher rates of leukemia in kids who ate 12 or more hot dogs per month. Antioxidants from vitamins A, C, and E when consumed at the same time may offer protection against cancer-causing effects of nitrosamines. The U.S. government requires meat packers to add ascorbic acid (vitamin C) to meats with nitrates for this reason. If your children eat food with nitrates, have them eat or drink something high in vitamin C at the same time.

One other source of nitrates in the food supply is in our water systems. Rural areas that use high-nitrogen fertilizers, especially those that are on well water, are most at risk. People in these areas should consider getting their water screened for this, especially if there are pregnant women or infants in the home. Use bottled water for babies under eight months of age if you have concerns about nitrates in your water supply.

For infants under about eight months of age, nitrates can have an effect on the hemoglobin that carries oxygen in the blood cells. Nitrates will convert to nitrites and this form reacts with the hemoglobin in the blood and causes "blue baby syndrome," or *methemoglobinemia*, a condition characterized by lack of oxygen in the blood. Infants may appear healthy, but show blueness around the mouth and feet and hands (newborns often have blue feet and hands in the first few weeks on and off because of poor circulation—this is not a problem). Nitrates are banned from baby foods because of this recognized toxicity. Other symptoms of nitrate toxicity in older children and adults can include difficulty breathing, dizziness, headaches, nausea, and vomiting.

Foods with nitrates should be given sparingly to children. Look for nitrate-free meats and hot dogs in the freezer section. I have discovered that my local grocery store "deli" section carries some luncheon meats without nitrates. However, you need to ask. Vegetarian hot dogs made from soy protein do not contain nitrates. Should you stress out if your child is at a birthday party and eats hot dogs? I would say relax, try to make sure they are taking in some extra vitamin C foods that day, and continue to control things you can in the home.

Water Contamination

Recent news is being made about levels of the cancer-causing toxin arsenic in our water system and what the government should allow as a "safe" level. The EPA has recommended lowering the allowable levels from 50 parts per billion (ppb) to 5 ppb in drinking water. Arsenic occurs naturally in rocks, soil, water, and air. Most areas of the United States have very low levels, but there are areas of "hot spots." The National Academy of Sciences states that the current standard could result in 1 person in 100 developing cancer over a lifetime of exposure. Government action is pending.

Water contaminants can include bacteria, viruses, and protozoa. One protozoa that many people have heard of is Giardia, which has caused periodic outbreaks of infections. Chemical contaminants are another concern. Chlorine by-products as a result of disinfection, lead, cadmium, mercury, nitrates (see previous section), radon, and pesticides are all identified in water systems. The U.S. Geological Survey has estimated that 15 percent of wells in agricultural and urban areas have nitrate levels above the EPA standard and that pesticides contaminated 54 percent of sample from wells and springs.[33] All may have negative health effects at high concentrations. The groups that are at highest risk for exposures to these toxins are infants, children, pregnant women, the elderly, and those who are immunocompromised.

Bottled water may not be any better than tap water. The Natural Resources Defense Council sampled 1,000 bottles of water from 103 brands and found that one-third had at least one bottle that violated state or industry limits for contaminants.

Further Information on Safe Drinking Water

EPA's Safe Water Drinking Water Hotline: (800) 426-4791 or www.epa.gov/safewater. Can direct you to a qualified lab for water testing and let you know what tests are appropriate for your area.

Natural Resources Defense Council: www.nrdc.org Report called "Bottled Water: Pure Drink or Pure Hype" with test results.

NSF International: (800) 673-8010 or www.nsf.org To find out about water filters standards.

How to Decrease Risks of Environmental Toxins

We obviously cannot control everything in our environment. However, when children are young, it is probably best to eliminate the few things we can control. Below are some measures that can be taken to protect your children from some of the risks of various toxins:

- **Buy organic foods when possible.** If your child is at a stage where he eats a lot of one or two fruits or vegetables, choose the organic variety more often. Organic baby foods can be purchased (Earth's Best, Gerber's Tender Harvest, Well-Fed Baby) or you can make your own baby food with organic produce (see p. 92, "Homemade Foods"). Another way to think of choosing organic foods is to note that chemical pesticides accumulate in fatty and oily foods. It is more important to look for organically labeled foods in cooking oils, butter, and nuts, especially peanuts. Look for organic peanut butter and make sure that it is not made with hydrogenated fats and oils. (See p. 55, "Fats: The Good, the Bad, and the Ugly.") Even with organic fruits and vegetables, wash them before serving. (See Appendix VI, "Organic Foods and Nutritional Products.")

Organic Foods
Labeling, Cost, and Nutritional Value

Labeling: National guidelines by the USDA are being established to ensure a consistent standard for organic labeling. Up until now, labeling has varied and has not been nationally standardized or regulated. Consumers will start to notice new organic labeling on products and full implementation of the guidelines will be in place by mid-2002. Some of the guidelines to be certified organic include:

- no chemical pesticides or fertilizers
- cannot be genetically modified
- cannot be irradiated
- organic livestock must be fed 100 percent organic feed
- no antibiotics in organic livestock
- sewage sludge from municipal waste water systems cannot be used as fertilizer for organically grown foods.

All agricultural products with the "organic" label must originate from farms or handling operations certified by a state or private agency accredited by the USDA. In addition, a product labeled "Made With Organic Ingredients," must have at least 70 percent of its ingredients from organic materials.

Cost: Cost can be an objection to the use of organic foods. *Consumer Reports* in January 1998 showed that although they are usually more expensive than conventional foods, there was some overlap in price. The cheapest organic produce was less expensive than the most expensive conventional produce. The organic industry is growing and pricing and availability will most likely improve. In looking at the big picture, is it worth it to pay a few pennies more for safer food that may decrease risky exposures for our family—and especially for our children?

Nutritional Value and Taste: Many factors influence the outcome for nutritional value and taste of a food. Being "organic" does not guarantee better taste or more vitamins or minerals. One argument for organic foods' better taste is that they must be sent to market as close to harvest as possible.

It may be hard for some families to choose or find organic foods. If organic produce is not readily available or out of your budget, at least consider taking the following measures:

- **Peel foods to remove some toxic residue.** Wash foods that cannot be peeled with diluted dishwashing detergent to help remove toxins. This should be done if they are organically grown or not. In the same Consumer Reports article, washing fruits and vegetables in this way eliminated pesticide residues in 53 percent of the produce tested. There are also special fruit and vegetable washes now available. Use a brush if necessary under running water. Remove outer leaves of leafy vegetables.

- **Look for non-GMO foods.** If you want to ensure that you are not buying GE foods in the United States, you will have to buy organic or look for labeling that says the product was grown without GMOs (genetically modified organisms). Cereals are one large source of GE foods for children. Healthier cereal brands that are labeled without GMOs include EnviroKidz cereals, Arrowhead Mills, and New Morning.

- **Use foods that are less likely to be contaminated.** In the Consumer Reports article, lower risks of contamination were found in apple juice, bananas, broccoli, canned peaches, milk, orange juice, and canned or frozen peas and corn. (See p. 38, "Less Contaminated Substitute Foods.")

- **Buy produce in season.** Produce out of season is more likely to be imported and shipped long distances. Food shipped long distances is more likely to be treated with post-harvest pesticides.

- **Buy locally grown foods.** Local food will be fresher, closer to ripeness, and more likely to have fewer pesticides and additives, since spoilage doesn't need to be retarded. Many farmer's markets will feature foods from organic farmers. You may also be able to find a food co-op that uses organic produce. These usually deliver or you can pick up once or twice a week in season, locally grown, pesticide-free foods.

- **Eat a variety of foods.** Rotating food choices will help reduce the risks of exposure to a food that has a lot of one chemical. This may be more difficult with "picky eater" type kids. Choosing organic for the "one-fruit" child may be safer.

- **Minimize the use of pesticides around the house,** particularly if you are pregnant or have small children. Store pesticides safely so that children cannot have access to them. Use pest control services only when necessary, and hire companies that use integrated pest management, which focuses on the least toxic methods. Make sure they are certified in your state.

- **Be aware of drinking water contamination.** To check for contamination, contact your local water supplier. This agency is required to have information on contaminants in your local water supply available to the public. You may want to consider a home water distiller or filter system. The filtration system must be checked periodically, and the filters must be changed as recommended. The EPA Drinking Water Hotline can help find a certified lab in your area to test your water. (See p. 34, "Further Information on Safe Drinking Water.")

- **Eat fewer animal products.** Because of concerns about hormones and antibiotics in meat, moderate meat consumption may be desirable, especially red meats and fatty cuts of meat. Since pesticides tend to concentrate in fat, trim all visible fat from meat and trim fat and skin from poultry. Dioxin is found in high concentrations in beef and pork. It is also found in higher concentration in higher fat dairy products, so using non-fat skim products is safer.

- **Limit or eliminate fish consumption while pregnant.** Because of the issues around mercury in predatory fish and PCBs from areas with water pollution, my opinion is to limit or eliminate fish consumption if you are thinking of getting pregnant or already pregnant. I would recommend not eating the high-risk fish mentioned in the "Mercury" section (p. 31). If you have concerns about fish or seafood, the FDA has a 24-hour FDA Seafood Hotline at 1-888-SAFEFOOD.

- **Choose organic milk and dairy products.** Certified organic milk means that the animals are fed 100 percent organic feed and that growth hormone and antibiotics should not be used. Organic milk and other dairy products (like yogurt, cheese, cream cheese, and butter) are more available now and can be found in many large chain supermarkets. In choosing organic dairy products, there appears to be clear advantages and no disadvantage other than cost.

- **Limit foods with nitrates.** Use foods with nitrates and, for that matter, with all other preservatives sparingly. Use healthier alternatives like vegetarian hot dogs, fresh cooked chicken rather than luncheon meats, nitrate-free hot dogs (available frozen, Shelton's is one brand), or meats. Encourage eating foods or drinks with a lot of vitamin C if your child does eat a food with nitrates.

- **Give your child a nutritional supplement.** Antioxidants found in vitamin and mineral supplements help to neutralize extra free radicals that may form as a result of environmental toxins. Read on to find out more about this in the next chapter.

Less Contaminated Substitute Foods

To reduce health risks if organic produce is not available, the Environmental Working Group recommends avoiding highly pesticide-contaminated food and choosing foods that are less likely to be contaminated. The foods listed under "Instead of these..." were most likely to be contaminated with pesticides and are ranked from higher to lower contamination risks. Foods listed under "Try these..." are less likely to have higher doses of pesticide contamination.[34]

Instead of these . . .	Try these . . .
strawberries	avocados
bell peppers	corn
spinach	onions
U.S. cherries	sweet potatoes
peaches	cauliflower
Mexican cantaloupe	Brussels sprouts
celery	U.S. grapes
apples	bananas
apricots	plums
green beans	green onions
Chilean grapes	watermelon
cucumbers	broccoli

Chapter Two

roundup

The Environmental Bad Guys

- Buy organic foods when possible.
- Wash and peel fruits and vegetables.
- Buy organic milk.
- Limit meat products and nitrates.
- Minimize home pesticide use.
- Check drinking water sources for contamination.
- Use a nutritional supplement for added protection.

Chapter Three
The Antioxidant Good Guys

Is the medical community doing everything it can to learn about nutritional health and inform their patients of what they know? Or are they waiting for all the research data to absolutely confirm what is appearing in the medical literature?

The official view from the medical community remains that our diet should be adequate to fulfill our nutritional requirements. Health officials claim there is no evidence that our current food supply is inadequate or lacking in nutrients or unsafe to eat. However, consumers are increasingly conscious of the link between nutrition and health, and many are concerned about the safety and nutritional value of the food they eat. Scientific information is accumulating in the adult medical research about the benefits of nutritional supplementation and natural remedies to prevent and treat diseases. Unfortunately, less research appears in pediatric literature. Those of us who treat children must use information in adult literature and extrapolate and restudy the information for children.

Our first efforts as parents must be directed at changing the dietary habits of our children and our families. Study after study shows that our children are not getting the nutrition they need. However, as caring parents, there will be phases and stages of frustration as we try to do the best for our children. Nutritional supplementation can be that extra insurance to protect their cells, but it should not be used as an excuse to feed "bad" foods to our children. If this is your attitude, please put this book down right now and re-examine your goals. Then, try to change one thing today to improve your family's diet and continue to implement changes gradually. To understand the role of supplementation and how it can protect against disease now and in the future, read on.

RDAs and Changes for the New Millennium

In 1941, the Recommended Dietary Allowances (RDAs) were developed to prevent diseases like scurvy (vitamin C deficiency) and rickets (vitamin D deficiency) and to maintain normal nutritional adequacy. Scientific evidence is mounting to show that intakes above the RDA can reduce the risk of chronic diseases. The RDA is not intended to determine safety standards. New standards are being developed with four reference points for nutritional adequacy, including the RDAs. The points are known collectively as **Dietary Reference Intakes (DRI)**. These include:

- **Estimated average requirement (EAR)** is the intake that meets the estimated nutrient need of 50 percent of individuals in a specific group.

- **RDAs** are the intake levels that are adequate to maintain the nutrient requirements of *nearly all* healthy individuals of a specific age and gender.

- **Adequate intake (AI)** is expressed for a nutrient instead of an RDA when there is not enough information to set the RDA. Nutrients for infants are often expressed in these values. (This is because studies are not done on infants, which may deprive them of life-giving nutrients.)

- **Tolerable upper intake level (UL)** is the maximum level of daily nutrient intake that is unlikely to pose adverse health effects to almost all individuals.

These new definitions should help those of us directing nutritional supplementation to understand how to provide amounts that are beneficial for health and to stay within safe limits.

Why Children Need Supplementation

As we saw in Chapter 1, poor dietary habits in children are the norm, not the exception. Children are often picky eaters, and because so many food choices are low in nutritional value, children are often eating the wrong foods. As discussed in the previous chapter, our children are being raised in a more challenging world, exposed to more toxins, pollution, and stress. They are exposed to free radical damage daily and in higher amounts than when their parents and grandparents were being raised. Air pollution, water pollution, pesticides, sun exposure, preservatives, radiation, smoke, excess exercise, fatty foods, and stress are factors that raise free radical levels. These free radicals increase risks of degenerative diseases as they cause cellular and tissue damage within the body. There is a great need for diets rich in vitamins, minerals, and antioxidants to combat the free radical damage. Children receiving a diet rich in fruits and vegetables are better able to counteract the effects of the extra toxins they might face.

Another possible problem is the quality of nutrients in our food supply. Fruits and vegetables are shipped far distances, and even from other countries. Because of early harvesting practices used to ensure freshness of the foods when they arrive at the store, our foods are not allowed to attain their maximum nutritional value. Research shows that fruit picked green contains less vitamin C. Also vitamin C and other nutrient losses occur when produce is stored for long periods of time.

Potatoes can lose 60 to 70 percent of their vitamin C in storage.[35] In addition, foods vary in their nutritional value. Carrots can vary by 50-fold in the amount of vitamin A they contain. When you select carrots, you have no idea if you are picking the ones with more vitamin A in them. Also, certain nutrients are dependent on the soil where the food was raised. As an example, selenium is an important mineral that depends on the soil content. Certain areas of the United States and some countries like New Zealand and China have selenium-deficient soil.

Think about how most families plan their grocery shopping. One large shopping trip a week is typical. Fruits and vegetables bought at the start of the week lose nutritional value after sitting on the counter or in the refrigerator. Then, the food is cooked and loses more nutrients. By the time it is microwaved and served the next day as leftovers, the value has significantly deteriorated.

Physicians' Attitude on Supplementation

Scientific studies are emerging rapidly and are confirming the benefits of supplementation in maintaining health and preventing disease. Scientists and physicians are talking more about using supplementation. Dr. Godfrey Oakley, Jr., a physician at the Centers for Disease Control and Prevention, stated in an April 1998 editorial in the *New England Journal of Medicine* that:

> Since the mid-1970's, 25 percent of American adults have regularly consumed a multivitamin containing 400 micrograms of folic acid. The current evidence suggests that people who take such supplements are healthier, and so are their children who take nutritional supplements. This evidence raises the question of whether physicians and other health care professionals should recommend that all adults take a multivitamin daily.[36]

Dr. Ranjit Chandra of the Memorial University, Newfoundland, and the World Health Organization Center for Nutritional Immunology states:

> The era of nutrient supplements to promote health and reduce illness is here to stay. Some data suggests that a reduction in the incidence and duration of infection may also occur. In North America, a year's supply of micronutrient supplementation costs less than three visits to a physician and much less than hospitalization for one day.[37]

Dr. Annette Dickinson, who is the Director of Scientific and Regulatory Affairs for the Council of Responsible Nutrition stated, "For most people, a rational supplement program to obtain generous intakes of protective nutrients would include a multivitamin with folic acid plus additional supplements of vitamin E, vitamin C, and calcium."

And when it comes to physicians themselves, a survey by a high school student that was published in the *Journal of Cardiology* revealed that slightly more cardiologists take antioxidant vitamins than aspirin to prevent heart attacks. Forty-two percent of them take aspirin, while forty-four percent take vitamin E, vitamin C, or beta-carotene, alone or in combination. Thirty-seven percent of the physicians interviewed recommend antioxidants routinely to their patients with cardiovascular disease.[38]

Some doctors are concerned that people who use supplements will rely on them as a substitute for good nutrition. National surveys show that 40 to 50 percent of Americans use nutritional supplements. As a group, they are more motivated to improve their diets. They appear to have a more nutritious diet than the general population.[39]

Medicine is slow to change positions. The medical community wants to see extensive research before recommending new drugs and therapies. Two examples in pediatrics demonstrate how medical opinion has been slow to change:

- Fifty years ago breastfeeding was not widely accepted by the medical community. Formula was thought to be the better choice for infants. Medical research took years to demonstrate the immense health benefits of breast milk.

- In the 1960's, researchers first suspected that folate, when taken by the pregnant mother, played a role in preventing neural tube birth defects. It wasn't until 1992, some 30 years later, that the United States Public Health Service recommended that all women who might become pregnant take a daily dose of 400 micrograms of folate.

Another reason for slow progress in the area of nutritional supplementation research is funding for research efforts. Pharmaceutical companies are better able to promote research efforts, where vitamin and supplement companies do not have these same resources.

Impact of Nutrient Deficiencies on Our Children

All the attention has been primarily on the adults, but our children also need these benefits. Research that has focused on the nutritional needs of children is summarized below.

- A poor childhood diet may make the brain more vulnerable to the risks of Alzheimer's. A group of elderly men who lived in Hawaii and had experienced poor, malnourished childhoods in Japan were studied. Short adult height was linked to poor nutrition, and it was found that those adults with the shortest stature had the highest prevalence of Alzheimer's.[40]

- Zinc supplementation reduces the incidence of acute lower respiratory infections. A study from India showed that children who were deficient in zinc and who were then supplemented with 10 milligrams of zinc had a 45 percent reduction in the incidence of pneumonia.[41]

- High levels of choline during pregnancy may enhance memory and learning capacity in the fetus. The National Academy of Sciences has designated choline an essential nutrient. Pregnant women should take 450 milligrams per day and nursing women should get 550 milligrams daily. Initial studies done with pregnant rats suggest choline supplementation may have long-lasting effects on brain function. Pups born to mothers that received no choline did poorly on tests designed to measure attention and certain types of memory.[42]

We are just starting to understand the role of certain nutrients in improving the health of children. Because of what is appearing in adult literature about supplementation decreasing the risks of heart disease and cancer, we need to take a serious look at supplementation for children. Could we further decrease risks of heart disease and cancer if children were given a nutritional supplement early in life? This information will take many more years to gather, but it is critical information for the future of our children.

Nutritional Supplementation in the First Year of Life

Pediatricians may prescribe a liquid vitamin with fluoride for this age group. The following gives information on some nutrient deficiencies infants may acquire during their first year.

Vitamin D

Vitamin D is a hormone that is formed in the body by a chemical reaction with sunlight. Breast milk contains very little vitamin D. Infant formulas and commercial milk are fortified with vitamin D. The other source of vitamin D is sunlight. *Rickets* is a rare bone disease of children caused by vitamin D deficiency. It is characterized by a softening of the bone structure. There are some inborn metabolic diseases that will cause rickets because of a problem in the way a child absorbs or processes vitamin D. Vitamin D deficiency may occur in breastfed babies who get little sun exposure. If you live in an area that has limited sunlight or where cold weather limits sun exposure, your baby may need a vitamin D supplement. Children living in areas with air pollution and haze were found to have lower vitamin D levels than children living in rural areas. Ask your pediatrician about vitamin D supplementation if your baby is breastfed and:

- you live in an area with little sun exposure
- your baby does not go outside, and
- your baby has very dark skin.

Fluoride

Fluoride is important for the enamel of the teeth and makes them more resistant to cavities; however, too much fluoride may cause a discoloration of the teeth called *fluorosis*. If you are breastfeeding, your infant may receive little fluoride from the breast milk even if the community water contains extra fluoride. Ready-to-feed and concentrate formulas, especially soy formulas, contain fluoride. If you are using powdered formula and tap water, your baby may be receiving enough fluoride. Home reverse osmosis systems will remove fluoride out of tap water, but carbon filters will not. Some bottled waters are available with extra fluoride.

Dental researchers analyzed the fluoride concentration of ready-to-eat infant foods and found that baby foods had a wide range of fluoride concentrations. Cereals, fruits, and vegetables had the lowest levels, while ready-to-eat foods with chicken had the highest levels. Researchers caution that babies receiving a diet with more than a couple of ounces of chicken a day may be at risk for receiving too much fluoride, especially if they are getting fluoride from other sources. Fluoride from other foods varied widely depending on the fluoridation of the water used in processing.[43] Discuss fluoride supplementation with your doctor to find out what is necessary for your area and situation. Fluoride is only available by prescription from a physician.

Tips For Healthy Teeth

- As soon as teeth erupt, wipe them with a washcloth daily.

- After a year of age, encourage regular tooth brushing before bedtime. Allow your baby to try brushing his own teeth and then take a few strokes across the surfaces yourself. Start flossing as early as possible (around 2 to 3 years of age for most kids), especially if the teeth are close together.

- Never use fluoridated toothpastes if your child is swallowing the toothpaste. Wait until children are old enough to spit it out, or use toothpaste that does not contain fluoride. If they swallow significant amounts of fluoride toothpaste, they may get fluorosis. A wet toothbrush is all you really need, but non-fluoridated toothpastes are also available.

- Don't allow a baby to routinely fall asleep with a bottle or while breastfeeding. After the teeth emerge, these babies will be at risk for developing serious tooth decay, known as nursing-bottle caries. Saliva production decreases at night, and any sugars from formula, breast milk, or juice will not be washed away and cavities will develop.

- Sugars promote bacteria overgrowth that produces acid and then causes tooth decay. Avoid a lot of dried fruits, candy, soda or juice in the diet. The fats in aged cheeses (e.g., cheddar and Swiss) seem to neutralize the bacterial acids and may help to decrease cavity formation. Xylitol, which is a natural sweetener in fruits and vegetables and in some brands of chewing gum, has also been found to decrease cavity production.

The following chart gives the current fluoride recommendations from the American Academy of Pediatric Dentistry and the American Academy of Pediatrics. Fluoride supplementation is based on the fluoride concentration in the local water system.

Fluoride Recommendations

age	less than 0.3 ppm of fluoride	more than 0.3 ppm of fluoride	0.6 ppm of fluoride
0 to 6 months	0	0	0
6 months to 3 years	0.25 mg	0	0
3 to 6 years	0.50 mg	0.25 mg	0
6 years up to at least 16 years	1.0 mg	0.50 mg	0

Fluoride concentration in the local water supply in parts per million – talk to your physician, dentist, or call your local water supplier to find out the concentration for your area.

Iron

Iron deficiency is the most common nutritional deficiency in the United States, usually found in older infants and young children under about three years of age. Lack of iron may cause a low red blood cell count known as anemia. With a significantly low blood count, children can be fatigued and pale. However, with a mild anemia, there may be very little outward signs, but prolonged iron deficiency can affect growth and impair the development and intelligence of an infant or child. The damage done in early childhood can be permanent. Studies have shown decrease in IQ, poor attention span, and poor social behavior as a result of iron deficiency.

The child's physician generally does screening tests for anemia at about nine to twelve months of age. Two servings of four tablespoons each of dry rice cereal will provide about 14 mg of iron. This will decrease the risk of iron deficiency anemia by 50 percent in the breastfed infants.[44] Early introduction of regular cow's milk (which contains no iron) before a year of age will increase the risk of iron deficiency. Babies born prematurely may begin life anemic and may need iron supplements early in life. These should be prescribed by a physician in a proper dosing.

Avoiding Iron Deficiency

Infants need iron. Use formula fortified with iron or breast milk until a year of age. Iron in breast milk (although present in small amounts) is well absorbed by the infant. However, babies deplete their iron stores after about four to six months of age (sooner in preterm infants or low-birth-weight infants). Therefore, iron foods should be introduced to babies who are exclusively breastfed after six months of age. Infant formulas are fortified with iron, and although less well absorbed than breast milk iron, it is generally enough to make up the difference.

Find iron foods to add to the diet. Some iron-rich foods include lean beef, eggs, fortified cereals and baby cereals, instant cream of wheat, spinach, dark green leafy vegetables, wheat germ, navy beans, egg noodles, blackstrap molasses, potatoes with the skin, soybeans, raisins, and prune juice. Animal sources of iron are better absorbed than plant sources of iron.

Cooking with iron foods. Add iron-rich grains to baked goods or combine with hamburger or meatloaf recipes. Grains such as quinoa flour and amaranth flour have good iron content. The raw grains can be cooked and added to soups, stir-fry dishes, or stuffing. (See p. 109, "Great Grains.") Add blackstrap molasses to recipes as a substitute for sugar, or add it to cereals or over pancakes and waffles.

Helping absorption of iron. Vitamin C containing foods aid the absorption of iron; milk and dairy products can decrease iron absorption by as much as 30 to 50 percent. So when children are eating their "iron foods" (more commonly at dinner), offer water instead with the meal and limit dairy if you find they need more iron in their diet. Children who consume excess amounts of dairy products can be at higher risk of iron deficiency anemia. For children between one and four years of age, total dairy intake of 16 to 24 ounces a day is plenty to meet calcium needs. If they are not taking iron sources of food, talk to your child's doctor about their risk of iron deficiency.

A word about supplementing with iron. Too much iron can be dangerous. Iron found in multivitamin supplements for children is generally considered safe when taken as directed and may need to be used for a child who does not consume foods with iron. However, if your child has been identified as having a significant iron deficiency anemia, a separate iron supplement may be necessary, but should only be taken under the direction of a doctor.

Accidental iron poisoning from iron-containing supplements is a leading cause of poisoning in the United States. Make sure to store iron supplements (even the adult brands with iron) safely away from children.

Nutritional Supplementation for Children Over One Year of Age

In my opinion, children over one year of age should be on nutritional supplementation. Fluoride supplementation depends on the fluoride exposure in the child's drinking water. If the child needs fluoride, ask for the prescription from your child's doctor or dentist as a separate fluoride only supplement. There is a prescription fluoride with vitamins, but it lacks minerals. By getting the fluoride alone by prescription, you can choose a broader multivitamin. Iron supplementation should be used if a child is anemic or if recommended by a physician because of poor iron intake in the diet. Iron, vitamin D, and fluoride supplementation needs will vary depending on the situation.

Nutritional supplementation with vitamins and minerals should be used **in addition** to offering a healthy diet. The principles of creating healthy eating habits that are outlined in this book should be the starting point.

So, how does a parent choose a nutritional supplement for children? The multitude of choices available at drug stores or health food stores can be overwhelming. One problem consumers face is that the dietary supplement industry is not strictly regulated. The Dietary Supplement Health and Education Act of 1994 (DSHEA) restricted the Food and Drug Administration's (FDA) authority over dietary supplements. The industry regulates supplements under food guidelines. There are no manufacturing or quality control testing requirements. As an example of lack of quality control, in September of 1998, *The Los Angeles Times* did a survey of ten brands of St. John's wort and found that seven had less active ingredients than was promised on the label.

The cheapest product is frequently not the best. Quality products often demand higher prices. Research the company by examining its web site, if available, or contact the company directly for information or literature. Check to see if the company has research scientists creating the product. Find out if the company follows Good Manufacturing Practices (GMP). One test is to ask the company to send you a copy of its "Certificate of GMP Compliance." A company that follows pharmaceutical guidelines for production is ideal. Look on the label and see if potency is guaranteed. This means that if you were to take this to an independent lab, the content of the product would match the label. Check the sugar and additive content of the vitamin. (See Appendix VI for suggested companies.)

A balance of vitamins and minerals should be offered to our children. Nutrients work synergistically, which means that certain vitamins and minerals work cooperatively in different metabolic pathways in our cells and tissues. Correcting a deficiency of only one vitamin may cause a deficiency in other areas. For example, excess vitamin B-1 can interfere with vitamin B-2 and B-6 and create deficiencies of these. The following highlights various vitamins and minerals and tells why they are necessary:

Vitamin A/Beta-carotene. Vitamin A is needed for growth and repair of body tissues, bone, skin, teeth, and hair. It is also important in maintaining the immune system. Carotenoids are compounds related to vitamin A, with beta-carotene being the best known of this group. When food or supplements with beta-carotene are consumed, the beta-carotene is converted to vitamin A in the liver. High doses of vitamin A supplementation can be toxic. No overdose can occur with beta-carotene, although if you take too much, your skin may turn slightly yellow-orange. I recommend using a product that contains beta-carotene, not vitamin A. Vitamin A deficiency is common in children living in underdeveloped countries. Although serious deficiencies are rare in the United States, young children and adolescents are apt to get less than the recommended amounts of vitamin A in their diet.

Vitamin C (ascorbic acid). Vitamin C is an antioxidant that helps with growth and tissue repair and is needed for healthy gums. It increases the absorption of iron. It works synergistically with vitamin E, and these two antioxidants are more powerful together than alone. Vitamin C is important in counteracting nitrosamines, a cancer-causing compound that is formed after eating cured meats containing nitrates. (See p. 33, "Nitrates.") Lower rates of cancer have been shown for those people with the highest vitamin C intake in their diet.

Vitamin D. Vitamin D aids in the absorption of calcium and phosphorus and helps build bone. It is necessary for normal growth and development of the teeth and bones in children. Most vitamin D comes from sun exposure. In adults, vitamin D deficiency will accelerate bone loss. Individuals who are obese have an increased risk of vitamin D deficiency.

Vitamin E. Vitamin E is now being recognized as an important antioxidant for reducing the risks of cancer and cardiovascular disease. It is necessary for tissue repair and promotes healthy skin, hair, nerves, and muscles. The current RDA for vitamin E in adults is 22 IU (International Units). Dosages of vitamin E necessary to decrease risks of cardiovascular disease and cancer are much higher than the RDA for vitamin E in adults. Dosages cited in research studies are often in the range of 100 to 600 IU.

Thiamin (vitamin B-1). Thiamine assists in blood formation, carbohydrate metabolism, and brain function. It is needed for transmission of impulses in the central nervous system.

Riboflavin (vitamin B-2). Riboflavin is used in red blood cell formation, antibody production, and aids in the metabolism of all foods. It also helps maintain normal vision. Research in animals showed that riboflavin-deprived animals had a high rate of cataracts. Research in animals also revealed that a lack of riboflavin during pregnancy caused birth defects.

Niacin (vitamin B-3, niacinamide, nicotinic acid). Niacin is necessary for metabolizing food, and aids in the function of the nervous system. The "niacin flush" (redness of the skin) can occur from dilated blood vessels with doses as low as 75 milligrams of nicotinic acid in adults. The flush is harmless and disappears within 30 minutes. Niacinamide, the form found in many supplements, does not cause flushing.

Pantothenic Acid (vitamin B-5). Known as the "anti-stress vitamin," pantothenic acid is involved in the manufacturing of adrenal hormones, antibodies, and neurotransmitters. It also helps in the breakdown and utilization of foods and vitamins.

Pyridoxine (vitamin B-6). Pyridoxine is necessary for the metabolism of proteins and carbohydrates. It promotes red blood cell formation and is needed for nervous system function.

Vitamin B-12 (cobalamin). Vitamin B-12 is required by cells to build the genetic material, DNA, and to form red blood cells. This vitamin is also necessary to prevent anemia. It is linked to the production of acetylcholine, which is a neurotransmitter. Strict vegetarians and those with gastrointestinal disorders that produce an inability to absorb vitamin B-12 are at risk for deficiency.

Biotin. Biotin assists in cell growth, fatty acid production, and in the metabolism of carbohydrates, fats, and proteins. It is necessary for the utilization of other B vitamins.

Folic acid (folate, folacin). Folic acid functions as a coenzyme in DNA and RNA synthesis, so it is necessary for cell growth and division. Folic acid has been found to be very important during pregnancy to prevent neural tube defects. It must be taken before conception and during pregnancy. Folic acid at high levels is nontoxic, but concerns have been raised about high intakes masking vitamin B-12 deficiency and pernicious anemia, which is caused by B-12 deficiency. This effect is apparent at intakes of 5 milligrams or more. Most experts agree that 1,000 micrograms (1 milligram) of folic acid per day plus food folates are without identifiable risks or side effects.

Calcium. Calcium is needed for strong bones and teeth. It also is important for maintenance of a regular heartbeat and for transmission of nerve impulses. It is needed for muscle growth and contraction. Calcium is critical for bone growth and bone mineralization in children. Dietary deficiencies of calcium may place our aging population at higher risk for osteoporosis. Although some foods are high in calcium, they may also be high in oxalic acid. Oxalates interfere with calcium absorption. High oxalic acid foods include almonds, beets, cashews, chard, green beans, kale, rhubarb, soybeans, and spinach. The best sources of calcium are dairy products. (See Appendix III, "Calcium Requirements and Foods.") Different forms of calcium are absorbed differently. Calcium citrate is better absorbed than calcium carbonate.

Chromium. Chromium is involved in the metabolism of glucose and in the proper utilization of insulin. The average American diet is deficient in chromium. Some evidence is appearing that links low chromium to diabetes; however, this evidence is not yet well established. Low chromium has also been linked to a higher rate of heart disease.

Iodine. A trace amount of iodine is important for a healthy thyroid gland and prevention of goiter. Iodine deficiency in children may cause mental retardation. Since the introduction of iodized salt, iodine deficiency is rare.

Magnesium. Magnesium is a catalyst in our body's enzyme activity. Magnesium, together with the proper balance of calcium, is necessary to promote bone mineralization. It is important for the transmission of nerve and muscle impulses. A deficiency of magnesium affects the metabolism of calcium, potassium, and sodium. Magnesium deficiencies have been linked to cardiovascular problems. Magnesium deficiencies are common in the American diet, especially in teenagers, women, and the elderly. The so-called "Type-A" personalities have been found to have low levels of magnesium.

Manganese. Small amounts of manganese are needed for protein, fat, and blood sugar metabolism. It is also necessary for healthy nerves and for a healthy immune system.

Molybdenum. This is needed for metabolism of DNA and RNA within the cells. People with diets high in refined and processed foods are at risk for deficiency.

Selenium. Selenium is a necessary co-factor for antioxidant enzymes that protect the immune system by neutralizing free radicals. Selenium deficiency has been linked to cancer and heart disease. Studies have also shown that 200 micrograms per day of selenium can significantly reduce the risk of certain cancers. Selenium works with vitamin E, and if you are deficient in selenium, the potential harm from vitamin E deficiency is increased. The selenium content in food is dependent on the selenium content of the soil where the food is grown.

Zinc. Zinc is important for enzyme systems in the body. It promotes a healthy immune system and speeds wound healing. It is needed for normal taste and smell, prostate gland function, growth, and sexual maturation. Mild, subclinical zinc deficiency is a common phenomenon. It is estimated that 48 percent of the world population is at risk of zinc deficiency. Zinc deficiency is especially common in children and women. The ability to absorb zinc declines with age. Marginal zinc deficiency in children can cause poor appetite, poor growth, and impaired taste. Breastfeeding mothers who are zinc deficient may pass on zinc deficiency to their infants. The zinc found in breast milk is better absorbed than zinc found in formula, even though there are similar levels. Zinc levels are lowered by diarrhea and fiber consumption and a significant amount of zinc is lost in perspiration. Compounds in grains and legumes, called *phytates*, bind with zinc so that it cannot be absorbed. Zinc deficiency is known to impair the immune system and make a person more susceptible to colds and infections. Studies in animal models have linked zinc deficiency with learning disabilities and poor attention span.

Signs of Deficiencies, Overdoses, and Food Sources for Vitamin and Minerals

The following chart provides information about signs of vitamin and mineral deficiencies, overdoses, and food sources for these vitamins and minerals.

VITAMIN	SIGNS OF DEFICIENCY	SIGNS OF OVERDOSE	FOOD SOURCES
Vitamin A	Night blindness; dry eyes; growth delay in children; dry skin; fatigue; frequent colds and infections	Abdominal pain; dry, itchy skin; hair loss; liver damage; blurry vision; headaches; joint pain *NOAEL: 10,000 IU	Dairy products, animal livers, green and yellow fruits and vegetables: apricots, asparagus, broccoli, carrots, papaya, peaches, pumpkin, red peppers, spinach, sweet potatoes, Swiss chard, squash
Vitamin C (ascorbic acid)	Bleeding gums; loose teeth; slow healing; easy bruising; dry skin; scurvy with above symptoms plus swelling, weakness, and pinpoint bruising under the skin	May cause kidney stones in those prone to stone development; diarrhea NOAEL: more than 1,000 mg (perhaps as high as 10,000 mg)	Citrus fruits, asparagus, avocados, broccoli, Brussels sprouts, cantaloupe, mangos, papayas, green peas, spinach, strawberries, tomatoes
Vitamin D	Rickets in children/ osteomalacia in adults (weakening and bowing of the bones); osteoporosis in adults	High blood pressure; high cholesterol; diarrhea; headache; fatigue; calcium deposits NOAEL: 800 IU	Fish oils, dairy products, egg yolks, liver, oatmeal, tuna, exposure to sunlight on the skin
Vitamin E	Damage to red blood cells; destruction of nerves; anemia and eye damage in premature infants	Bleeding; consult a physician if you are taking an anticoagulant medication (blood thinner) NOAEL: 1,200 IU	Dark, green, leafy vegetables; legumes, nuts, seeds, wheat germ, brown rice, cornmeal, corn oil, soybeans, liver, egg yolk
Thiamine (vitamin B-1)	Constipation; fatigue; irritability; loss of appetite; muscle wasting; beriberi in severe cases with above symptoms plus possible nerve damage	Too much of one B vitamin may cause a deficiency of other B vitamins NOAEL: 50 mg	Asparagus, broccoli, brown rice, egg yolks, fish, legumes, liver; most nuts, plums, prunes, pork, poultry, raisins, wheat germ, whole grains
Riboflavin (vitamin B-2)	Cracks and sores at the corners of the mouth; dermatitis; hair loss; insomnia; light sensitivity; poor appetite	Very safe at high doses NOAEL: 200 mg	Asparagus, avocados, broccoli, dairy products, fish, kelp, leafy greens

* NOAEL (No Observed Adverse Effect Level): NOAEL is the intake level where there are no credibly substantiated adverse reactions noted in adults. Adapted from the Council for Responsible Nutrition: *Vitamin and Mineral Safety - A Summary Review.*

mcg = micrograms   mg = milligrams   IU = International Units

VITAMIN	SIGNS OF DEFICIENCY	SIGNS OF OVERDOSE	FOOD SOURCES
Niacin (vitamin B-3)	Canker sores in mouth; diarrhea; dizziness; pellagra in severe cases; dermatitis, diarrhea, depression	Liver damage; ulcers; irregular heartbeat; rashes; high blood sugar NOAEL: 500 mg nicotinic acid; 1,500 mg as nicotinamide	Beef liver, broccoli, carrots, cheese, dates, eggs, fish, milk, peanuts, potatoes, tomatoes, wheat germ, whole wheat products
Pantothenic Acid (vitamin B-5)	Unknown in humans	Diarrhea; water retention NOAEL: 1,000 mg	Beef, eggs, fresh vegetables, legumes, liver, nuts, pork, whole wheat
Pyridoxine (vitamin B-6)	Seizures, weight loss, vomiting and irritability in infants; glossitis (inflammation of the tongue), cracks at the corners of the mouth, depression, itchy, dry skin in adults	Sensory neuropathy with loss of feeling in hands and feet NOAEL: 200 mg	All foods contain some B-6, but foods with the highest amounts are carrots, chicken, eggs, fish, meat, peas, spinach, sunflower seeds, walnuts, and wheat germ
Vitamin B-12 (cobalamin)	Anemia, neurological damage; deficiency can occur in strict vegetarians who eat no animal foods	Can occur in infants with a rare genetic disorder NOAEL: 3,000 mcg	Dairy products, eggs, meats, poultry, seafood
Biotin	Rare, except in infants, where it may cause "cradle cap," a dry scaly scalp; dry skin; fatigue; insomnia; loss of appetite	None described NOAEL: 2,500 mcg	Brewer's yeast, egg yolks, meat, milk, poultry, saltwater fish, soybeans, whole grains
Folic Acid (folate, folacin)	Anemia; digestive disturbances; fatigue; memory problems; insomnia; irritability	Megadoses can mask vitamin B-12 deficiency and interfere with zinc absorption NOAEL: 1,000 mcg	Barley, bran, brown rice, cheese, fortified cereals, green leafy vegetables, legumes, meats, milk, mushrooms, oranges, wheat germ, whole wheat
Calcium	Rickets in children; osteomalacia in adults (weakening and bowing of the bones); osteoporosis in adults; brittle nails, eczema, heart palpitations, muscle cramps	Kidney stones; calcium deposits in tissues; muscle and abdominal pain; interferes with absorption of zinc and iron NOAEL: 1,500 mg	Almonds, broccoli, dairy products, salmon (with bones), seafood, soy products, tofu, green leafy vegetables

VITAMIN	SIGNS OF DEFICIENCY	SIGNS OF OVERDOSE	FOOD SOURCES
Chromium	Anxiety; fatigue; imparied glucose tolerance	No adverse effects from chromium from food sources or dietary supplement sources. NOAEL: 1,000 mcg	Beer, brewer's yeast, brown rice, cheese, meat, mushrooms, oysters, potatoes, prunes, rhubarb, whole grains
Iodine	Goiter (large thyroid gland); mental retardation in children	Sores in mouth; metallic taste; diarrhea; vomiting NOAEL: 1,000 mcg	Iodized salt, seafood, kelp
Magnesium	Muscle weakness and cramps; disturbances of heart rhythms	Diarrhea NOAEL: 700 mg	Dairy products, fish, meat, nuts, peanut butter, tofu, green vegetables, watermelon, whole wheat
Manganese	Not known in humans	Nerve damage NOAEL: 10 mg	Avocados, nuts and seeds, seaweed, whole grains
Molybdenum	Not known in humans	Joint pain resembling gout	Beans, cereal grains, legumes, peas, dark leafy vegetables
Selenium	Anemia; fatigue; sterility	Brittle nails; fatigue; gastrointestinal disorders; hair loss; irritability NOAEL: 200 mcg	Meat and grains, but dependent on the soil where the food is raised
Zinc	Slow wound healing; loss of appetite; delayed growth and sexual development in children; loss of taste and smell; white spots on fingernails; impotence; dull hair	Nausea; vomiting; gastric bleeding NOAEL: 30 mg	Beef, cheese, lentils, oysters, peanuts, pecans, pine nuts, pork, turkey, wheat germ, whole-grain cereals

Fats: The Good, the Bad, and the Ugly

Why include a section on fats in the chapter on antioxidants? Because fats have a good side and these good fats can be considered a necessary part of a healthy diet and supplementation program. This section will provide a general overview of the benefits of good fats and the ugly side of bad fats. Despite all the concern about fat in our diet, the body does require fat to function. The problem is that most people are getting the wrong kinds of fats in their diets. Children under two years of age should **not** be on a low-fat diet. For infants under a year, most of their fat should be from formula and breast milk. The total fat concentration of formulas and breast milk is around 45 to 50 percent of their total calories. Over two years of age, children start to approach adult recommendations of less than 30 percent total calories from fat and less than 10 percent from saturated fat. There are two types of fats:

- The bad guys: *Saturated fats* are the type that can clog arteries. These fats are usually solid at room temperature and are in meat, milk, and poultry. However, tropical oils like palm oil, palm kernel oil, and coconut oil are liquid at room temperature and are saturated fats. High intakes of these fats have a correlation with an increased incidence of heart disease and strokes.

  Trans fats, often listed as hydrogenated oils, are found in margarines, vegetable shortening, and many processed foods such as in peanut butter, chips, cakes, cookies, crackers, and fried fast food. New studies show these may be more dangerous to health than saturated fats.

- The good guys: *Unsaturated fatty acids* are liquid or soft at room temperature. The two main categories are *monounsaturated fats (MUFAs)* and *polyunsaturated fats (PUFAs)*. The fatty acids that are necessary for the body and cannot be made by the body are called *essential fatty acids* (EFA). Essential fatty acids are part of the good fats that have been researched and found to have numerous health benefits. (See p. 59, "EFA: Benefits and Sources.") Essential fatty acids help build nervous system tissue and help with the transmission of nerve impulses. They are also used by the body for the production of *prostaglandins*, hormone-like substances that regulate various processes.

FATS TO AVOID

Foods Usually High in Trans Fats* (avoid the words "hydrogenated" or "partially hydrogenated")		Foods High in Saturated Fats
biscuits	fried fast foods	coconut oil
cakes	margarine *(esp. those with coconut, palm kernel, and hydrogenated oils)*	lard
candy bars		shortening
some cereals		
cinnamon rolls	muffins	
cookies	some peanut butter	
corn chips	pies	
doughnuts	potato chips	

*Usually these are foods that are packaged and boxed in stores.

UNSATURATED FATS

Monosaturated Fats	Polyunsaturated Fats (EFAs)	
	Omega-3 Fats	Omega-6 Fats
avocado oil	canola oil*	borage oil
canola oil*	fish oil	corn oil
high oleic safflower oil	flaxseed oil	cottonseed oil
high oleic sunflower oil	soybean oil**	grapeseed oil
olive oil	walnut oil	peanut oil
		primrose oil
		safflower oil
		seasame oil
*canola oil is high in both **MUFA** and **PUFA**	soybean oil**	
** soybean oil is high in both omega-3 and omega-6 fatty acids	sunflower oil	

There are two major categories of EFAs, which are both polyunsaturated fatty acids (PUFA). These are **omega-3** and **omega-6** fats.

- The omega-3 fats include alpha-linolenic acid, eicosapentaenoic acid (EPA) and docosahexaenoic acid (DHA). Omega-3 EFAs are found in fresh oily fish (canning causes some loss of EFA) like herring, mackerel, salmon, tuna, and anchovy. Flaxseeds, omega-3 enriched eggs, and walnuts also contain omega-3 fats.

- The omega-6 fats include linoleic acid, gamma-linolenic acid (GLA), and arachidonic acid (AA). These fats are found in common vegetable oils found in the chart above.

Getting an adequate amount and proper ratios of essential fatty acids may present a challenge. The Western diet has moved away from a fish diet, and most of the fats in processed foods are the bad fats. Also, consider that if your child does not get adequate amounts of the basic vitamins and minerals, his or her body may not process the EFAs that are consumed. In order for EFAs to be used correctly, they need certain co-factors such as vitamins A, C, and E and minerals such as magnesium, selenium, zinc, and copper.

The primary problem is that the Western diet tends to be too high in omega-6 and too low in omega-3 fatty acid consumption. The typical American diet has a ratio of omega-6 to omega-3 of around 15 to 1. Diets with a ratio of about 4 to 1 have been shown to be healthier in research studies. One important study, known as the Lyon Diet Heart Study, looked at heart attack survivors. Three different diets were assigned: a traditional heart diet, the "prudent" heart diet (recommended by the American Heart Association), and a modified version of the Crete diet.[45] This last diet group received a ratio of omega-6 to omega-3 of 4 to 1. Two years into the study, the study was stopped because survival rates of the Crete diet were so significant compared to the other two diet groups. There was a 76 percent lower risk of dying from a cardiovascular event with the Crete diet. Also, laboratory animals that received a diet high in omega-6 fatty acids and low in omega-3 fatty acids had more invasive and faster growing tumors when implanted with cancer cells. Psychological tests found these animals also suffered with more difficulty through mazes and had more random behaviors. Signs of essential fatty acid deficiency include excess thirst, frequent urination, dry hair, dry skin, dandruff, and small hard flesh-colored bumps (called keratosis pilaris) on the arms and thighs.

If everything is working correctly, EFAs along with their co-factors will become metabolized into prostaglandins in the body. These are important in the function of the immune system. Too much saturated fat can block the conversion of EFA to these desirable prostaglandins. A malfunctioning immune system can lead to illness, and it also plays a role in allergies and autoimmune diseases (diseases like inflammatory bowel disease, juvenile diabetes, and juvenile rheumatoid arthritis). The use of EFAs to improve allergies, asthma, and attention deficit disorder is addressed in Section C of this book.

Baby Fats for the Brain

The adult brain is about 2 percent of total body weight and uses 20 percent of total energy. The fetal brain is about 16 percent or more of body weight, uses about 70 percent of energy for growth, and is made of about 60 percent fat. The brain triples in size from birth to age one. The fats required for the nerves found in the brain are primarily DHA and AA. Since breast milk is made of 40 to 50 percent fat, we see how Mother Nature built in the right components for brain development.

Investigators are discovering the importance of different fats on infant brain development. How these fats affect attention, problem-solving ability, IQ, and visual function is the emphasis or recent research. Consider these studies:

- DHA appears to be important for visual development in premature infants.[46]

- A study from Australia showed that supplementation of infant formulas with a dietary omega-3 did improve visual function to the level of those found in breastfed infants.[47]

- Another study showed that supplementation of formula with PUFA from birth to 4 months of age resulted in higher problem-solving scores at 10 months of age.[48]

- People with neurologic problems such as depression and attention deficit disorder have shown improvements with omega-3 supplementation.

- The improved intelligence and academic performance of breastfed babies compared to formula-fed babies has been partially explained by the increased DHA content of breast milk.

- A study from the *British Medical Journal* showed that patients with multiple sclerosis were less likely than controls to have been breastfed for a prolonged period of time.[49]

If you are pregnant, or breastfeeding, you should make sure you are including EFAs in your diet. The amount of EFAs in the breast milk is dependent on the mother's diet. I prefer the plant-based forms of omega-3 fats or supplements that are screened for toxins rather than fish, because of the risks with toxins in fish. (See box below, "Fish Caution.") My recommendations are one tablespoon of flaxseed oil and a fish oil supplement with DHA and EPA. The total omega-3 as fish oil (DHA plus EPA) should total about one gram a day. I recommend both because you receive the proper balance of omega-6 and omega-3 in the flaxseed oil. Also, the flaxseed oil has the precursor to make the AA, which as previously mentioned, is also an important part of the fats in infant brain.

If your baby is formula-fed, you should note that formulas contain some essential fatty acids, but not in the same amounts or of the same varieties as found in breast milk. The most important fats, DHA and AA, have not been approved for use in infant formulas in the United States. The British Nutrition Foundation and the World Health Organization have recommended the use of DHA in infant formulas and these fats are added to formulas in over 50 countries around the world. Blood levels of DHA have been shown to be lower in formula-fed infants than breastfed infants. Hopefully, addition of these nutrients to U.S. infant formulas will occur in the near future.

Infants and children can safely take essential fatty acids in the form of flaxseed oil. See the box below on "Essential Fatty Acids: Benefits and Sources" to find ways to add good fats to your child's diet.

Fish Caution
During Pregnancy or With Breastfeeding

Remember the section on mercury toxicity in Chapter 2. (See p. 31) Pregnant and breastfeeding women should be cautious of adding fish into their diets, especially freshwater fish from polluted waters with PCB's and dioxin or predatory fish such as shark, swordfish, and tuna. Recommendations currently are to eat the predatory fish no more than once a month while pregnant, but my opinion is to prevent extra risks on infant brain development and avoid fish altogether during this crucial time. Damage done during this period is irreversible. Fish oil supplements may seem safer, but some fish oil supplements are contaminated with pesticides and heavy metals such as mercury. Check with the supplement company to see if they screen for this and ask for documentation from the company. One company that does meet high standards for their fish oil capsules is USANA (see Appendix VI for ordering information). They guarantee their BiOmega-3 capsules to be free of heavy metals, organic contaminants, pesticides, and trans-fatty acids.

Essential Fatty Acids:
Benefits and Sources

Possible health benefits of essential fatty acids

- Lowers serum cholesterol and triglyceride levels

- Lowers blood pressure

- Lowers the risk of heart disease and death from heart disease

- Improves symptoms in rheumatoid arthritis patients

- Reduces the frequency and severity of migraine headaches

- Improves vision, especially night vision

- May help prevent and arrest growth of breast, colon, prostate, and pancreatic cancers

- Possibly lowers the risk of autoimmune diseases like multiple sclerosis, rheumatoid arthritis, and diabetes

- Improves skin conditions, such as eczema and psoriasis (see Chapter 13)

- Improves lung function of asthmatics (see Chapter 13)

- May be beneficial for children with attention deficit disorder (see Chapter 15)

Essential fatty acid supplements (see Appendix VI for sources)

- Flaxseed oil. This is an excellent source of omega-3 (as alpha-linolenic acid) and omega-6 fatty acids. It must be refrigerated. Do not cook with this oil as cooking destroys the fatty acid. Mix with foods like yogurt or smoothies. Sprinkle over cooked pasta, vegetables, or mix as part of salad dressings.

- Fish oil capsules. A source of omega-3 fatty acids with the all important DHA and EPA.

Food sources of omega-3

- Use canola oil (look for "cold-pressed" or "unrefined" canola oils, which have more antioxidants and flavonoids) or olive oil (extra-virgin olive oil has more omega-3 and the least omega-6) in recipes that require vegetable oil. Canola oil should be refrigerated.

- Free-range eggs contain more omega-3 fatty acids than the usual supermarket eggs. There are also omega-3 enriched eggs available at health food stores and some regular grocery stores.

- Flaxseeds or flaxmeal (ground flaxseeds) can be sprinkled on cereals, yogurt, or salads and added to the batter of breads, muffins, pancakes, and cakes. They should be refrigerated or frozen.

- Buy canola oil mayonnaise.

- Walnuts are rich in omega-3 fats and contain 90 percent unsaturated fats.

- Fish with essential fats include fresh tuna, salmon, mackerel, flounder, sardines, trout, anchovies, and herring. Fish that has been farmed is lower in omega-3 fatty acids because they are not fed a natural diet.

- Good sources of both omega-3 and omega-6 are Great Northern beans, kidney beans, navy beans, soybeans, and soybean oil. Soybeans (the Japanese call these "edamame") are now readily available fresh or frozen at health food stores and many regular supermarkets.

Chapter Three
roundup
The Antioxidant Good Guys

- Our children are exposed to a world very different from the world 50 years ago with more toxins and potential for free radical damage.

- Numerous studies confirm the health benefits of proper nutrition and nutritional supplementation in adults; benefits for children are also being discovered.

- In the first year of life, vitamin D, fluoride, and iron supplements may be necessary. Fluoride and iron may be needed beyond the first year of life. These supplements should be discussed with your child's physician.

- Make sure to include omega-3 sources in the maternal diet when breastfeeding.

- Find food sources or supplement infants and children with omega-3 sources. Look for signs of EFA deficiency and add EFA sources into the diet.

- Look for a reputable nutritional company.

- Our children will most likely receive both long- and short-term benefits from nutritional supplementation.

SECTION

B

Nourishing Kids the Best Way Possible

Chapter Four
Infants: Birth to Four Months

The gift of life at the moment of birth is remarkable, awe-inspiring, and scary. This fragile baby, a part of our being, is a dependent soul and will rely on us for protection, love, and feeding. Feeding, as all new parents discover, is one of the most time-consuming parts of caring for a baby. This precious baby doesn't just sleep sweetly and languish in your kisses and love, but cries, wails, and demands being fed just as you are wishing for some sleep yourself. Oh, so tiny. Oh, so fragile. Oh, so dependent on us. That is the scary part. How can we adequately feed and protect this little one who has come into our lives?

Fortunately, babies are the easiest group to offer food because of their natural instinct to eat. Babies root, suck, and swallow; cry when hungry; and relax when full. Parents get to decide whether to feed the infant with human milk or formula. This choice seems easy after we look ahead and see all the other daily eating choices available to our toddlers through adolescents and how they can become picky eaters. Most babies are not picky at this stage (thank goodness!). However, some babies will do better with some milk types than others. The main problem with babies is they are tiring because they believe the restaurant is always open.

The most important decision is whether to breastfeed or formula-feed. Starting your baby out right with a positive feeding experience takes patience and an understanding of usual feeding patterns for babies. There are some babies who develop difficult behaviors, like colic, spitting up, and snacking. These problems, and their solutions, will also be discussed in this chapter.

Human Milk Vs. Formulas

If you are truly concerned about the long-term health effects of nutrition on your child, there is only one right answer when asked whether you should choose human milk or formula. Extensive research has shown the health benefits of human milk, which include nutritional, immunological, psychological, social, developmental, environmental, and economic benefits.

A woman who is unable to initiate or continue to breastfeed because of lack of information or support should be a thing of the past. There are many community resources available through hospitals and private lactation consultants who provide women with breastfeeding support. It is amazing how one simple change in technique can bring success to a mother who thought she was doomed to fail. Seek help if you need it! It is very rare that a woman with proper support cannot manage to establish breastfeeding. (See Appendix V, "Breastfeeding Resources.")

If you are still trying to decide about breastfeeding, consider the following advantages of breast milk.

- **Health benefits.** Human milk contains antibodies and white cells that help fight infections including diarrhea, respiratory infections, ear infections, urinary tract infections, blood infections, and infections in the fluid around the brain (meningitis). Infections in breastfed babies may be less severe. Human milk may have a possible protective effect against sudden infant death syndrome, diabetes mellitus, asthma, Crohn's disease, ulcerative colitis, other chronic digestive diseases, and lymphoma. There are also studies that show that children who are breastfed have better intellectual skills and educational achievement that persists into young adulthood.[50]

- **Bioavailability of nutrients.** Human milk is something that cannot be exactly duplicated in any formula. Formula companies are constantly trying to search for the perfect human milk substitute. Many trace factors have yet to be understood or even discovered in human milk. The colostrum, which is the first milk after birth, is rich in vitamins and nutrients and has a special laxative effect that allows the baby to get rid of meconium, his or her first stools. Minerals such as iron and zinc are in breast milk in a form that is better absorbed than what is found in formula. Human milk composition varies from woman to woman, within a feed, over a day, and over time. These variations can never be duplicated in a formula.

- **May delay or decrease the severity of allergies.** Human milk rarely causes allergic reactions in newborns. If allergic symptoms do appear, first look at the maternal diet and eliminate common allergens like dairy products, eggs, nuts, or soy. There is evidence that prolonged exclusive breastfeeding will reduce the incidence of food allergy and intolerance, even if there is a strong family history of allergies. Breastfeeding may also delay the onset or decrease the severity of allergies.[51 52 53]

- **Easily digested, rarely constipates.** Human milk is a natural laxative and breastfed babies rarely get constipated. Constipation with hard stools is more often a problem for formula-fed babies. Breastfed babies will sometimes develop an infrequent stool pattern after two months of age, and they may only have a stool once every three to seven days. The stool is soft, and usually there is a lot of it, often requiring a full bath. If your breastfed baby is under a month of age and having infrequent stools, please check with your doctor and make sure that the infant is gaining weight well. *Infrequent stools from a breastfeeding baby under a month of age may be an indication that he or she is not getting enough milk.*

- **Convenience and low cost.** Human milk does not need to be heated or prepared. You never run out or have to go to the store in the middle of the night. It is ready to serve and is just the right temperature. There is usually enough for your baby, and there can be no mistakes in preparing human milk. It is free, except for the equipment purchased like nursing bras, pads, and pumps.

- **Bonding.** The maternal-infant bonding with breastfeeding is very strong. This does not mean that a bottle-fed baby cannot develop a healthy maternal-infant bond, but breastfeeding seems to make it easier to develop that bond. Hormones are produced in the nursing mother that promote a strong physiologic bonding between her and infant. Some studies have shown that breastfeeding mothers secrete endorphins, which are substances that lead to feelings of well being.

- **Exposes the child to a variety of flavors.** The flavor of breast milk is dependent on the maternal diet, and as the mother's diet varies, the baby becomes exposed to a wider variety of flavors. This may allow the child to adapt to new foods and flavors later in life.[54]

- **Fewer tendencies to overfeed.** Often with bottle-feeding, the tendency is to have the baby finish the full bottle. With breastfeeding, the right amount should be always available, and there is less of a temptation to overfeed. Overfeeding can contribute to more risk for obesity later in life.

- **Benefits for the mother.** Breastfeeding reduces the chances of maternal hemorrhage after birth. When the newborn suckles on the breast, this causes a release of a hormone called *oxytocin* in the mother, which helps the uterine muscles contract and decreases the risk of heavy bleeding. Oxytocin also helps the uterus return to normal size faster. Because breastfeeding uses up fat reserves, weight loss can be easier when breastfeeding. Breastfeeding burns about 250 calories per day. Some studies have shown that breastfeeding may produce a protective effect against developing breast cancer, ovarian cancer, and hip fractures later in life.

How Long to Breastfeed

The American Academy of Pediatrics recommends breastfeeding until the infant is a year of age. For women who are juggling a work schedule or attending to other children, pumping and using expressed breast milk has become easier. With newer and more efficient breast pumps on the market, pumping is more convenient. In the first eight weeks of life, the baby has an immature immune system and infections in this time period are potentially serious. Every attempt to give breast milk during this crucial time is ideal.

After six months, babies are expanding their food choices to include more solids. Breast milk is less of a focus in their diet after six months. Some women may choose to explore a combination of breastfeeding and formula supplementation. This can be done and is more beneficial than not breastfeeding at all. I would strongly urge breastfeeding up to a year whenever possible.

Getting Enough Milk

The first few days. This is every parent's concern, especially with the breastfed baby. If breasts had ounce marks, it would be a lot easier! In the first day or two of life, formula babies often take only ½ to 1 ounce or so at a feeding and then work up to 2 to 3 ounces in a bottle. This is probably a similar volume that the breastfed baby receives in colostrum at the first feedings. Then, as the milk comes in after 2 or 3 days, the baby will be taking more volume. In the first few days, all babies tend to lose weight, and they may lose up to 7 to 10 percent of their birth weight in the first few days. For example, an 8-pound baby may lose 9 to 12 ounces in the first 3 or 4 days. Over 10 percent weight loss, and the baby may be at risk of dehydration. By 2 weeks of age they should be back up to birth weight. Try to nurse at least 7 to 8 times in the first 24 hours and more if demanded by the baby. Expect some cluster feeds where the baby may feed every ½ hour to an hour for a short time and then take a longer sleep stretch of 4 hours. In the first few days, mothers are encouraged to try to awaken their babies to feed if it has been longer than 3 or 4 hours. At least 1 meconium stool (this is the baby's first stool, which is dark and tarry appearing) should occur in the first 48 hours of life and 1 wet diaper should occur in the first 24 hours of life. By day 3, breastfed infants typically have 3 to 4 wet diapers and 1 to 2 stools that are turning green to yellow in color.

Four days to four weeks of age. Breast milk is usually "in" by three to five days of age. You should be able to hear the baby gulping and swallowing during nursing and the baby should seem calm after breastfeeding. The baby should last two to three hours before the next feeding during some parts of the day. Stools should be changing to the loose, yellow mustard-color stools and the baby should be having at least three to four substantial stools a day. Urination (pale yellow) should be frequent enough for six diaper changes a day. Some babies can have up to eight or ten stools a day, often after every feeding. *If a baby is under four weeks and not having this type of stool or urine pattern, this could indicate that baby is not getting enough milk. Have the baby seen by a physician.* Bottle-fed babies should be taking three to four ounces of formula about every three to four hours by the end of the four weeks, or around twenty to twenty-eight ounces a day. Weight gain is another good indicator of adequate intake and is usually around one to two ounces a day.

Order Dr. Wood's Newborn Care and Feeding
audio tapes at
www.kidseatgreat.com.

Supplemental Bottles

Presented below are some of the few rare health reasons that breastfeeding may not be recommended or may be difficult.

- There is a rare woman who physically cannot establish an adequate milk supply. Women who have had prior breast surgery may have difficulty with their milk supply. Breast augmentation usually does not affect lactation, where as breast reduction is a more invasive surgery that may have an adverse affect on lactation.

- Women with certain infectious diseases may be counseled not to breastfeed. Women with the AIDS virus, HTLV-1 (human T-cell leukemia virus type 1), or active, untreated tuberculosis are counseled against breastfeeding. Most other diseases should not be a problem for breastfeeding, but should be discussed individually with a physician. Some diseases may require a temporary discontinuation, but pumping can keep up milk supply until the situation is safe for the baby.

- There are a few rare metabolic diseases (e.g., galactosemia) where infants cannot receive breast milk. Babies with these diseases cannot break down certain components in the breast milk and can become very ill. Babies with some metabolic problems, such as phenylketonuria (PKU), can breastfeed and supplement with a special formula as long as they are being closely monitored.

- Certain medications that a mother has to take may pass into the breast milk and cause problems for the infant. Anyone taking drugs of abuse (such as marijuana, cocaine, or heroin) should not breastfeed. Some temporary medications may require a temporary discontinuation of breastfeeding. While on a temporary medication, the mother can pump to maintain the milk supply and discard the milk. Then when she has discontinued the medication and it is safe to breastfeed, she can resume breastfeeding. Medications that must be continued for the nursing mother and have potential side effects for the baby may require that the mother permanently stop breastfeeding. Most over-the-counter medications are safe while breastfeeding, but always check with your doctor. If you are nursing and you need to take any type of prescription, non-prescription, herbal, or natural remedy, consult with your physician.

- There is a very rare baby that refuses to "latch-on" and nurse, despite support from the best lactation specialists. Premature babies or babies with oral-motor problems such as cleft palate, may have a harder time with breastfeeding. In these situations, pumping and giving the breast milk in a bottle can be an option and can be carried out as long as the mother can keep up her milk supply and is willing to keep pumping regularly.

If you are breastfeeding and choose to introduce a supplemental bottle, try to wait until at least three to four weeks of age when breastfeeding should be well established, and the baby should be gaining weight well. The exception is when directed by a lactation consultant or physician because of medical issues or poor weight gain. If extra milk is needed in the first few weeks, try to use a lactation aid, like a dropper or syringe, for feeding and not a bottle. Hopefully, this will eliminate the problem of "nipple confusion" where the baby finds bottle-feeding easier and refuses to breastfeed.

If you are choosing to use supplemental bottles with formula, make sure breastfeeding is well established and decide when and how often you will choose to supplement with formula. The more formula bottles used, the less demand for breast milk, and this will reduce milk supply. Discuss your formula choice with your infant's doctor. If you are thinking of changing formula for some reason, this should also be discussed with the doctor. Consider the following options when examining formulas:

- **Milk-based formulas.** Popular milk-based formula brands include *Similac, Enfamil,* and *Carnation Good Start.* The milk protein in formula is modified and is less allergenic than regular cow's milk. The American Academy of Pediatrics sees no role for the use of low-iron formulas in infant feeding and only recommends the use of high-iron formulas. Formula-fed infants need extra iron. Babies tolerate the high-iron formulas as well as the low-iron formulas, and iron is not thought to be the cause of constipation or intestinal distress.

- **Soy-based formulas.** These brands include *Isomil, Prosobee,* and *Alsoy* formula. These are made from a soy protein. Some babies tolerate these formulas better than the milk-based formulas. They can be used in some infants who have an allergy to the milk-based formulas. However, some infants with more serious types of allergic reactions to cow's milk (like blood in the stool) may do better using the hydrolysate formulas listed below. Infants who are allergic to a milk-based formula may also be allergic to the soy protein. (See p. 74, "Facts on Food Allergies.")

- **Lactose-free formulas.** *Lactofree* is the infant formula marketed specifically as lactose-free. *Isomil* and *Prosobee* are also lactose-free. True lactose intolerance is rare in infants and usually shows up in children over three or four years of age. Lactose intolerance can cause gassiness and diarrhea. Sometimes lactose-free formula is suitable if an infant has a diarrhea infection, because he or she temporarily loses the ability to break down lactose with many of the viral and bacterial intestinal infections.

- **Hydrolysate formulas (hypoallergenic).** The proteins in these formulas have been broken into smaller pieces (hydrolyzed) so they are less likely to induce allergic reactions than the previously listed formulas. *Nutramigen, Alimentum,* and *Pregestimil* are three choices that are recommended if a baby has symptoms of being allergic or intolerant to the milk and soy formulas. These formulas are more expensive than the regular formulas—about three times the price. Babies who have been on milk or soy formula for a while may refuse these special formulas because they taste so different. Talk to your baby's doctor if you are having difficulty getting your baby to accept the new formula. One other formula, *Neocate,* is an elemental formula that is used for babies who cannot tolerate any of the others or who have severe symptoms of milk protein allergy.

- **Follow-up formulas.** These are marketed to target babies over six months of age. It is not necessary to make the switch to these if your baby is doing well on one of the formulas above. A few are designed for children over a year of age. Formula is not necessary over a year old and the switch to regular milk will be made then.

- **Organic formula.** Currently, there is a new organic formula on the market, called *Baby's Only Organic Formula.* The manufacturer has a dairy-based and a soy-based option for the formulas. It is available at health food stores and some grocery stores. Caloric and nutritional information is available on the company's web site at www.naturesone.com. Because this is a newer formula, testing and experience is not as extensive as the other choices and should be used with the approval of the baby's doctor. I would suggest you print out the nutritional information or bring the label for the doctor and let him or her review it.

- **Don't use goat's milk, regular cow's milk, or homemade formulas for infants.** Goat's milk and cow's milk fail to meet the recommended daily intake for vitamins and minerals as established by the Food and Nutrition Board Institute. Lack of iron in these milks raises the risk of iron deficiency anemia. Homemade formulas with evaporated milk or other combinations should not be given. Despite some of the limitations, commercial baby formulas are still the best choice if the baby cannot breastfeed.

Baby Fat and Beyond

We don't worry about fat babies and thunder thighs in this age group! Baby fat present at this age does not mean babies will have a weight problem later on. Studies suggest that breastfeeding offers protection against later obesity. After a year of age, many children become pickier eaters and often consume a smaller amount of food. Babies start to thin out once they begin crawling and walking at about 9 to 15 months of age. However, if you have concerns or it appears that your baby is excessively hungry, discuss this with your physician.

Water, Juice, and Solids

Water is not necessary for newborns unless there is a medical problem. Some medical circumstances may require early supplementation with water or a rehydration fluid like *Pedialyte* or *Infalyte,* but this should be discussed with your doctor. Human milk or formula should be enough to keep your infant hydrated, provided he or she is getting enough of it.

Juices are absolutely not necessary for this age group! Juices have little nutritional value, are full of empty calories, and are mainly a sugar source. (See p. 102, "What's the Problem with Juice?") One juice that is sometimes recommended to relieve constipation is prune juice. Keep in mind that constipation with hard stools is more of a problem for formula-fed babies.

Solids should not be introduced until after the baby is four to six months old. Well-meaning grandparents are often the ones to question you about introducing solids prior to four months. Many raised their children with solids as early as a month or two of age. New evidence has emerged that early solids may be harmful because they may trigger more allergic responses, especially in babies where there is a family history of allergies. The intestinal tract absorbs large molecules with the solids that may later be recognized as foreign proteins and cause an allergic reaction. Developmentally, babies younger than four months are not ready to take solids with a spoon because they have a tongue thrust that prevents them from taking the food and swallowing it.

The early solids rule is occasionally broken for the baby who is spitting up excessively. The physician may recommend adding rice cereal directly into a bottle of formula or breast milk. This helps to thicken the feeding and allows the milk a better chance of staying down. This should be discussed with your doctor first.

The Breastfeeding Mother's Diet and Nutritional Supplementation

When you are nursing, particular attention must be paid to your diet and your nutritional supplementation. Toxins (like the nicotine from smoke, and illegal drugs) are passed onto your baby. Nicotine passes into the breast milk and decreases the amount of oxygen in the baby's blood. It also diminishes milk supply. These toxins should be avoided at all cost, otherwise it is best not to breastfeed.

Fluids. Fluids are very important, and nursing mothers tend to be thirsty. Drink to quench your thirst, but you do not need to flood yourself. Water is the best fluid. Make sure it is healthy water. (See p. 34, "Water Contamination.") Milk is not a necessary part of the diet to ensure healthy breast milk. Some babies may show signs of an allergy to the milk protein that crosses into the breast milk when the mother consumes dairy products. (See p. 74, "Symptoms of Food Allergies.") Intakes of highly acidic juices or foods (like oranges and grapefruits) by the mother may cause the baby to develop diaper rashes from the acidity.

Foods. When you are nursing, you are the food supply. Your milk is dependent on the intake of your nutrients. Eat a balanced diet with the recommended 30 percent of calories from fat. Lots of fresh fruits and vegetables will help boost antioxidant levels to help you stay healthy. Pollutants and toxins can pass into the milk supply. Try to vary foods to diminish exposure to the same toxins or pesticides commonly used on certain foods. Think about choosing organic foods to reduce exposure to pesticides for you and your baby. Avoid nitrates in foods (see p. 33, "Nitrates") and try to limit foods with colorings, artificial sweeteners, and MSG. Try to avoid high consumption of trans fatty acids, which cross into breast in breast milk and may interfere with the synthesis of the "good" essential fatty acids. Look for healthy sources of the "good" essential fats for your diet. (See p. 55, "Fats: The Good, the Bad, and the Ugly.") Limit or eliminate fish from the diet if you are breastfeeding because of the toxins currently found in fish. (See Chapter 2.)

A variety of flavors in the mother's diet will also expose the baby to different tastes. Flavors like garlic, vanilla, mint, and blue cheese are particularly transmissible. Studies suggest that experience with a variety of flavors during breastfeeding may make breastfed infants more willing to accept unfamiliar flavors than their formula-fed counterparts. Some foods can make your baby gassy and fussy. (See p. 73, "Is it Colic?")

Dieting while breastfeeding. This must be done sensibly. Strict diets for weight loss may affect milk supply and milk quality. Consider the following suggestions.

Weight Loss for the Nursing Mother

- You can diet sensibly while breastfeeding. Calorie intakes around 1,800 calories a day are considered safe and intakes lower than 1,500 calories a day are not recommended when breastfeeding. Wait until after the baby is about two months of age before attempting to diet, to allow time for your body to recover and to ensure that milk supply is adequate.

- Limit empty calorie junk food, processed foods, and refined sugar. The best rule is to follow signals for hunger and thirst, and follow the Food Guide Pyramid. Eat a balanced, varied diet and include foods that are rich in calcium, zinc, magnesium, vitamin B-6, and folate.

- If you are close to normal weight, one to two pounds per month of weight loss is suggested. If you are significantly overweight, your goal for weight loss should be around three to four pounds per month.

- Exercise is an important part of losing and maintaining weight loss. Although a few studies suggested that babies were less likely to take post-exercise milk (presumably because of slightly elevated levels of lactic acid), a review article on this issue concluded that it is not likely to be a problem in most cases.[55]

Continue taking your prenatal vitamin. Essential fatty acids are important for infant brain development, so take a supplement of EFAs, especially if you are on a lower fat diet.

Nutritional supplements. Nutritional supplements are just as important to nursing mothers as they are to pregnant women. (See Chapter 3 for a complete discussion of nutritional supplements.) There are some vitamins and minerals that are especially important to consume when breastfeeding.

- **Calcium.** Calcium intake is important to maintain while nursing. Recommendations from the National Academy of Sciences in 1997 state that all adults between 19 and 50 years of age should take 1,000 milligrams of calcium per day. They do not recommend that lactating women increase their daily calcium intake, but that lactating women consume levels that are appropriate for their age. It may not be possible to get this amount from diet alone, especially if your baby turns out to be sensitive or allergic to your dairy intake. (See Appendix III, "Calcium Requirements and Calcium Foods.")

- **Vitamin B.** The vitamin B content of breast milk is dependent on maternal intake of the B vitamins. Strict vegan mothers, who avoid all animal foods, including dairy and eggs, are at risk for producing milk that is deficient in vitamin B-12. Vegetarians in general are also at risk for producing milk that is low in zinc, iron, protein, riboflavin, and vitamin D. A deficiency of vitamin B-12 can lead to anemia, damage to the nervous system, and poor growth in the infant. Women who take high doses of vitamin B-6 (at levels greater than 200 milligrams a day) can suppress milk production.

- **Vitamin D.** The vitamin D content of human milk is also dependent on the maternal vitamin D intake. For mothers who avoid vitamin D-fortified foods, such as milk or cereal, and have limited exposure to sunlight, a vitamin D supplement should be taken. When exposure to sunlight is limited during cold weather seasons or when custom requires clothing that covers all of the skin, there is a possibility of both the mother and baby developing vitamin D deficiency. If the infant's exposure to sunlight appears to be inadequate, the infant should receive a vitamin D supplement.

Sun Safety

Protect babies with shade and clothing and avoid direct sunlight as much as possible. The American Academy of Pediatrics recognizes that when adequate clothing and shade are not available, parents can apply a minimal amount of sunscreen to small areas, such as the infant's face and the back of the hands. Babies do not need to wait until six months of age to use sunscreen. Studies show that sunscreen use does not interfere with vitamin D absorption.

- **Iron.** Some mothers need extra iron to battle anemia. Maternal iron supplements can upset the baby's stomach and cause gas and fussiness. Don't take iron supplements for a few days to help determine if iron is the cause of colic-type behavior. If your baby appears to have problems with the iron intake, discuss your options with your obstetrician before discontinuing the iron supplement.

- **Essential Fatty Acids.** Include omega-3 fat sources in your diet and/or as supplementation to help with infant brain development. (See p. 55, "Fats: The Good. the Bad, and the Ugly.")

See the Kids Eat Great web site for a
special report on prenatal nutrition at
www.kidseatgreat.com/prenatal.html

Problem Feeders

There are some situations that crop up in the newborn period that can be a challenge for a parent. I will touch on three common problems: colic, spitting up, and constant snacking. *The following sections discuss the baby who is over three or four weeks of age and who has seen the doctor and is gaining weight well without any other apparent medical problems.*

Is It Colic?

"Is it colic?" is the question I hear a few times a week from distraught parents. Colic describes the baby who goes through inconsolable crying spells and who does not respond to the usual comfort measures. The baby seems to have some type of abdominal discomfort, but there is no known cause. Most commonly, these episodes of crying occur at the same time of the day, usually in the evenings. Colic is every parent's fear, but fortunately, sometimes we can identify a real cause for the colic-type behavior. If you have ruled out these treatable causes, discussed below, you may just have the classic colic baby. If you suspect any of the following treatable causes apply to your baby, discuss them with your doctor.

If your baby is breastfed, consider some of these situations:

- **Food allergies vs. food sensitivities.** Some babies are sensitive to the foods you eat, or they may be truly allergic. There is a difference in these two problems, although some of the symptoms can look the same. *Food sensitivity or intolerance* causes gassiness, fussiness, or a change in stools. An example of food intolerance would be the diarrhea, cramping, and bloating that occurs with lactose intolerance. The person lacks the enzyme to digest lactose, a sugar found in milk. Food sensitivities can be caused by broccoli, cabbage, onions, beans, garlic, chocolate, or spicy foods. Excess caffeine has been known to cause irritability and colic-type behavior in some infants and can decrease the milk supply. Caffeine is found in chocolate, coffee, tea, and many soft drinks. Chocolate has a caffeine-like substance that can also cause a reaction. True *food allergies* may cause symptoms that are listed in the box below. A food allergy involves an immune system reaction where the body recognizes the food protein as foreign and creates an allergic reaction. It may take weeks, months, or even years for a food allergy to develop. It occurs after repeated exposure to the food and then the food finally triggers an allergic response. Dairy, peanuts, eggs, soy, fish, or shellfish are the food allergies most commonly seen. Wheat is less often identified as the culprit. If you suspect a food allergy, discuss it with your doctor. Additional tests are sometimes needed to help identify the offending food, and the potential seriousness of some food allergies needs to be discussed.

  If you are having difficulty identifying the food culprit for either a food sensitivity or a food allergy, eliminate the suspicious foods and then gradually reintroduce them one at a time. Occasionally, a small amount of a food is not a problem, but a large amount will cause your baby to have symptoms of the sensitivity or the allergy.

Symptoms of Food Allergies

- Chronic congestion, sneezing
- Hives, an itchy rash that looks like welts or insect bites
- Eczema, an itchy rash with dry, scaly patches; commonly seen on the face and creases behind the knees and elbows
- Vomiting shortly after the offending food
- Diarrhea, watery stools (for breastfed babies, since they are always loose, these are stools that are mostly water without any substance)
- Blood in the stool
- Gassiness, fussiness, colic behavior, or stomachaches
- Wheezing in the lungs
- Anaphylaxis is a rare, life-threatening allergic reaction that causes swelling in the mouth and throat, difficulty breathing, and eventually shock.

Facts on Food Allergies

Allergies tend to run in families, so if there is a family history of hay fever, asthma, eczema, or food allergies, you need to be more careful about introducing foods. Women who eliminate dairy products, eggs, fish, and peanuts from their diet during pregnancy and lactation may reduce the risk of their baby developing allergies in the first year of life. It is recommended that children at high risk for allergies (those with a family history) can also decrease their risk or delay the onset of allergies by:

- breastfeeding exclusively for at least the first six months or using a hypoallergenic formula
- delaying the introduction of solids until after five or six months of age
- delaying the introduction of cow's milk until age 1 or later, and eggs until age 2; peanuts, nuts, and fish until 3 years of age.

Cow's milk is the most common food allergy in children. About 70 to 80 percent will outgrow this allergy by about 3 or 4 years of age. Infants will need to be on a special hypoallergenic formula and a mother who is breastfeeding will need to eliminate dairy products from her diet.

Eggs are another common allergen. It is the egg white that is allergenic. Egg whites should not be given to infants under a year of age. If your child is allergic to eggs, he or she may develop an allergic reaction to the measles, mumps, rubella vaccine (MMR), and the flu vaccine. These vaccines are made with egg products. Check with your pediatrician if you have concerns about an egg allergy, when your child is due for these vaccines.

Wheat allergy is the most common type of grain allergy. Use wheat after seven to nine months of age and only after your child tolerates rice and oats. Wheat allergies tend to run in families, so if there is a family history of wheat allergies, delay wheat introduction further and try it cautiously.

Soy allergies can occur in infants and children. About half of children who are allergic to milk are also allergic to soy. Almost all those with soy allergy will outgrow it.

Peanuts can cause a very difficult allergy because even a slight exposure to the nut can trigger a reaction. Food that is even cooked with peanut oil can cause a serious reaction. Only about 20 percent of peanut-allergic children will outgrow their allergy.

Shellfish, berries (like strawberries and blackberries), and *chocolate* can cause allergic reactions. This usually first appears in older children, or even adults, who will claim they couldn't be allergic because they have been eating that particular food all their life. It can happen!

If your child does have a particular food allergy, you must pay attention to the ingredients listed in food labels. If he or she has a serious allergy, order a medical alert bracelet for your child. Allergy testing with blood work or skin tests may be necessary. Because of the seriousness of some allergic reactions, always discuss trying a known past allergen with your child's doctor before reintroducing it.

- **An overactive let-down reflex.** Some women suffer from too much milk that comes out very quickly. Their babies are chugging and gulping throughout the feeding. Milk sprays everything in sight if your baby accidentally pulls off. These babies are often gassy and fussy, gain weight quickly, have lots of wet diapers and stools, and want to nurse frequently. The suggestion for this situation is to try to have the baby nurse on one breast at a feeding. One let-down is better than two in this case and because the baby nurses so quickly, he or she has a better chance of getting the fattier, richer hind milk with just one breast. Also, use a position where the baby is lying more on top of you or sitting upright. This can be accomplished by leaning back in a nice comfortable chair, so the baby is sucking against gravity, or by using a football hold with the baby sitting upright. It is easier for the baby to control the flow if the milk is not squirting in the back of the throat. Simethicone drops (like *Mylicon*) are available over-the-counter and may be helpful to relieve gas. An occasional pumped bottle of expressed breast milk will help to give mother a break and the baby may be less gassy with a bottle because he or she can control the flow.

Case Report
An Overactive Let-Down Reflex

Justin was three weeks old when his mother, exhausted and in tears, came to my office for a lactation consultation. The baby was a pound and a half over his birth weight, so there was not a milk supply problem. He wanted to nurse every two hours and was fussy and passed a lot of gas. He had 10 to 12 stools per day. She had used simethicone drops, which helped some of the time. When the nursing was observed in the office, he was choking and gulping vigorously throughout the nursing. He pulled off several times and would cry and then get back to nursing. He only nursed for five minutes. He was not crying after the nursing, but squirmed and seemed uncomfortable. We talked about her overactive let-down reflex, which was causing him to choke, swallow air, feed quickly, and have more gas. I suggested positioning the baby so that he was lying more on top of her or side-lying nursing, nursing on one breast per feeding, and using an occasional bottle of pumped milk. The main thing was that she was relieved to find out that there was nothing wrong with him and was then able to relax about his feeding pattern. After six weeks of age, things were easier. He was nursing every three to four hours and was more comfortable.

- **Low milk supply.** At the end of the day, milk supply typically diminishes. Breastfed babies may be fussy and want to eat frequently at this time because they are hungry. One trick is to pump milk from the morning, when supply is usually higher, and save a top-off bottle for the evening. If your baby seems fussy and is snacking in the evenings, feed an extra ounce or two of breast milk in a bottle after you nurse (if over three or four weeks of age). Hopefully, the time until the next feeding will be longer and more milk will be available at the next feeding. If you have a baby who seems hungry and fussy all day long, have a weight check to make sure he is getting enough food and is not simply hungry.

- **Growth spurts.** Breastfed babies go through periodic growth spurts where they nurse more frequently for a day or two. This increases the mother's milk supply. The milk supply is based on supply and demand, so when your baby demands more, the supply will respond by increasing. It is best during growth spurts to follow your baby's signals and nurse frequently. This commonly occurs at two weeks, six to eight weeks, and three to four months of age.

If your baby is formula-fed, consider this situation:

- **Allergy or intolerance to the formula.** Occasionally, a baby will have an allergy to a formula. Review the allergy symptoms previously discussed. Babies may be allergic to cow's milk formulas, soy formulas, or both. About half of the babies who are allergic to milk will also be allergic to soy. Those infants allergic to both need to be on a hydrolyzed protein formula, like *Alimentum, Pregestimil,* or *Nutramigen.* If you suspect a problem with formula allergy or intolerance, please discuss this with your baby's doctor before making a change.

If your baby is either breastfed or formula-fed, consider these possibilities:

- **Stool infections.** Occasionally, a newborn may develop an infection with a bacterium or virus that may make him or her gassy or fussy. The stools may be watery and even contain blood or mucous. Remember that stools of breastfed babies are always loose and are about the consistency of mustard. If the stool is watery and mostly soaks into the diaper, this may be a sign of diarrhea. A stool culture will need to be obtained to make the diagnosis and decide if any treatment is necessary. Constant green stools may indicate hidden blood in the stool and shoud be tested by the doctor.

- **Swallowing excess air.** This condition can occur when a baby cries a lot, uses a pacifier, or gets air with bottle-feeding. Try to burp your baby frequently during feedings. Simethicone *(Mylicon)* drops may be used safely for the gassy baby. Different nipples or bottle systems may be helpful in reducing the excess air problem for bottle-fed babies. If the baby seems frustrated with taking the bottle, make sure the nipple holes are not clogged and see if the baby does better with a larger size nipple hole.

- **Spitting up.** Sometimes babies who spit up are fussy and have colic behavior. (See the next section for further details on this problem.)

If none of the above situations seem to apply, you may just have the classic "colic" baby. Realize that all babies do have fussy periods. There are babies who have a difficult temperament and require more attention. These babies need more cuddling and patience, and they often respond to different calming techniques such as swings, rocking, swaddling, music, warm baths, and car rides. Evening fussiness, which may be due to boredom, can be common. You will notice that when your baby is held for a few minutes, he will be fine but will become fussy again in a short time. If you change positioning or walk to a new environment, he will calm immediately, but will fuss again after a few minutes. You may go through this cycle several times in an hour. This is what I call "baby boredom."

Spitting Up

This is a common problem in babies. It is also known as *gastroesophageal reflux.* Mothers with babies who spit up are commonly found carrying around an assortment of "burp rags" and wearing washable cotton clothing. This problem occurs in babies because the muscle (called the *gastroesophageal sphincter*) located between the esophagus and the stomach is weak and ineffective at holding food down in the stomach. Spitting up may occur in small or large amounts and after some or all feedings.

If the baby is gaining weight well and is not fussy, there is no reason for concern. Babies may not outgrow this problem until a year old. Signs that may indicate more of a problem with gastroesophageal reflux condition are:

- Arching the back while feeding
- Pulling off the breast or bottle numerous times while feeding
- Excess fussiness during or after feedings
- Constant congestion (from irritation of milk into the nose, which may lead to ear infections)
- Wheezing (the baby may be aspirating food into the lungs)
- Poor weight gain.

The first three symptoms indicate that the baby may be having pain and irritation in the esophagus (heartburn or *reflux esophagitis*). The last three problems are some complications of excess spitting up. Any of the above signs should be discussed with your doctor. Medications or thickening the bottle feedings with rice cereal may need to be prescribed.

Measures that can be taken to help the baby who spits up include:

- Feeding the baby with the head raised above the body
- Burping frequently during the feeding
- Having the baby sit upright for 15 to 20 minutes after the feeding (an infant car seat is great for this purpose).

NOTE: Projectile vomiting is different from spitting up. Spitting oozes out or comes out with slight force, whereas projectile vomit would shoot across the room forcefully. Projectile vomiting may be a sign of a blockage in the intestinal tract (called *pyloric stenosis*). Consult your pediatrician as soon as possible if you see projectile vomiting.

The Snacker

This is the baby who is over two weeks of age and wants to feed every hour or two throughout the day and night. Babies can have a few cluster feedings scattered here or there, which may be normal. For the baby over two weeks old who eats constantly, feeding can quickly become a tiring and tedious job. *First, check with your doctor to make sure that your baby is gaining weight well and that there is nothing medically wrong with your baby. A nursing baby who is feeding very frequently and seems hungry all the time may not be getting enough breast milk.*

If the baby is bottle-fed, try to increase the amount in the bottle and see if the baby will feed longer at one time and go longer between feedings. The average baby at two weeks takes a three to four-ounce bottle. By two months, the baby may be up to four to six ounces, and then by four months the baby may take six to eight ounces per bottle. The average bottle-fed baby eats every three to four hours.

If the baby is breastfed, you should refer to the "Is it Colic?" section (p. 73). If none of those problems apply, your baby is snacking, your milk supply is adequate, and your baby is gaining weight, then you may just have a baby who is used to smaller, more frequent feedings. Frequent nursing can be a vicious cycle. The baby is snacking on a small volume of breast milk and is hungry an hour or two later. A top-off bottle of an ounce or two given immediately after nursing can be helpful. Before you consider starting a bottle, make sure your baby is over three or four weeks of age and is nursing well.

If you give a bottle with expressed breast milk right after breastfeeding, the baby may take the extra ounce or two and then go longer until the next nursing. This allows mom to create a little more milk for that next feeding. It may reduce the exhaustion level if this is leading to a decreased milk supply. One or two top-off bottles a day may do the trick. Usually, these are only needed for a few days.

Some babies love to nurse and snack for no good reason. Make sure you are recognizing the correct signals for hunger. Sometimes, parents become so involved with nursing to settle a slightly fussy baby that they forget that the baby may calm if held or given a little attention. At night, after two months of age, try to disregard the small noises and awakenings because sometimes you will see that your baby will go right back to sleep. However, if your baby is fully awake and crying, go ahead and feed. Most babies can start to sleep through the night by four to six months of age.

Great Eating Tips
for Newborns to Four Months

Whether you have chosen to breastfeed or bottle-feed, there are some steps that will encourage your baby to develop a positive attitude towards feeding.

- **Use a demand feeding schedule.** It is usually recommended to use an "on-demand" feeding schedule and not a strict feeding schedule. Sometimes, with a sleepy baby in the first few days of life, the infant needs to be prodded to awaken and eat every two or three hours. Once nursing is established and the doctor has checked your baby for adequate weight gain at the two-week check-up, you should be able to allow your baby to dictate the feeding frequency. The infant should be receiving six to eight feedings in a 24-hour period. Even formula-fed babies will have variations in their schedule and intake.

- **Observe your baby for signs of hunger and fullness.** Babies are all different in their signals for hunger and fullness. Positive feeding patterns can be created if a parent is sensitive to the baby's signals. Look for *feeding cues* such as squirming, fussing a little, moving the hand to the mouth, smacking the lips, and eye opening. Crying is often a late sign of hunger. Sometimes when a baby is very hungry and crying hysterically, it can be difficult for him or her to focus on eating. This is especially a problem for the breastfeeding baby who won't latch on because he or she is upset. Try allowing your baby to suck on your finger for a few minutes to calm and then latch your baby onto the breast. Watch for signs of your baby being full, which include falling asleep or taking only intermittent, weak sucks. If bottle-feeding, don't try to force the last ounce down just because you don't want to waste it. Remember, adults have an appetite that will vary, and so do babies!

- **Frequent feeding patterns.** Some babies who are feeding every hour or two after the first few weeks are giving cues other than just hunger. If you pick him up and he calms right away, try holding, bundling, walking around or playing with him instead of feeding right away. Just make sure the baby is gaining weight well to assure yourself he is getting enough milk. (See p. 79, "The Snacker.")

- **Understand different feeding temperaments.** Babies have different styles of feeding, and it is important not to let that frustrate you. Some babies are lazy feeders and are content to nibble at the breast or bottle. Others have a more vigorous style of feeding and seem to lust for food.

- **Do not force the nipple into the mouth.** Take advantage of your baby's natural rooting reflex, and brush the nipple (either breast or bottle) across the lips. Don't force or jam the nipple into the mouth.

- **Safe water.** Use filtered or distilled or boiled tap water water for babies during the first few months. You can boil water for at least five minutes. Consider having your water officially tested if you are planning to use tap water. (See p. 34, "Water Contamination.")

- **Bottle tips.** There is no one preferred nipple shape that infants will take; experiment and find what works for your baby. If the nipple hole is too large, the baby may be gulping too much milk, and if the hole is too small, the baby may seem frustrated and pull off the bottle a lot. It is best to warm the bottle of expressed breast milk or formula in a bowl of hot water for a few minutes or under tepid running water. Never prop the bottle or allow the baby to feed alone. Lying flat with bottle-feeding may increase the risk of ear infections. Discard bottles that have been partially eaten by the baby. Bacteria and enzymes from the saliva mix with the milk and a later feeding with the same bottle will be contaminated. You may sterilize bottles and nipples for their first use. After that, wash in very hot, soapy water or use the dishwasher. This is usually adequate for killing germs.

- **Breast milk storage tips.** Expressed breast milk can be refrigerated and used within 48 hours. Label frozen milk and store in the back of the freezer for as long as 3 to 4 months. After thawed, it should be used within 24 hours and not be refrozen. Microwaving can change the composition of breast milk and is not recommended.

- **Get fathers involved.** It is important for dad to be able to be involved with the bonding that occurs with feeding. Once the bottle has been successfully introduced, I "prescribe" a night of sleep for mom. Dad can do a late night or early morning feeding to give mom a longer stretch of sleep if she is breastfeeding. This can be done at any time along the way for the formula-fed infant.

- **Enjoy the feeding experience.** Women who maintain a positive feeding experience with their babies tend to have more success and less problem feeders. Babies can sense stress and anxiety in feeding, and this can lead to a negative feeding experience for the baby. Of course, we can't always lead a stress-free existence, but we need to try to stay relaxed while nursing. Try to limit potential distractions like the phone (that's what answering machines are for).

- **Talk calmly and quietly with your baby while feeding.** Put on soft music or do your own deep-breathing exercises. Make eye contact with your baby and observe how your baby reacts to your voice and your actions. Sometimes, when a mother is anxious about a baby who is not feeding well, the tendency is to jiggle her baby, the bottle, or the breast. This over activity may disrupt the baby's feeding. Imagine someone moving us around or moving our food around while we ate; it would not be a pleasant experience.

- **Loosen control.** For many mothers, the demands of fitting household chores, activities, and obligations to other family members into their schedule can be overwhelming. For women who are used to controlling their schedule, this loss of control and erratic feeding schedule can be distressing. Trying to take too much control of their baby's feeding pattern is unlikely to develop a positive feeding pattern. If the doctor feels the baby is doing well and gaining weight well, then relax. Let go of some control. So what if the dishes pile up or the house is messier than usual... enjoy this precious time.

Chapter Four
roundup
Infants: Birth to Four Months

- Carefully consider your choice of whether to breastfeed or give formula. It is an important decision!

- If you are breastfeeding, watch your diet and maintain a nutritional supplementation regimen. What you eat can affect your baby, both positively and negatively.

- Babies should be gaining weight at about an ounce per day for the first month.

- Be observant of your baby's signals for hunger and fullness and recognize that temperaments can vary.

- Don't allow yourself to get caught up in schedules and routines early on.

- Look for problem feeders and direct remedies to specific problems.

- Simply enjoy, enjoy, enjoy!

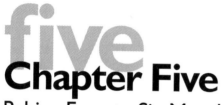

Chapter Five
Babies: Four to Six Months

The happy cherub seems to have arrived. Babies at this age are easy to entertain and seem to smile constantly. They are learning to reach and grab for everything in sight and of course, it all goes in the mouth. Toes are a favorite item to suck on—imagine that we were all so flexible at this time of our lives. Babies will vary in their readiness to start solids. Some may seem ready the second you place that first spoonful of food in their mouth, and some may scrunch up their face and act like you were feeding them lemons for lunch. Recognize when your baby is ready. By the end of this stage, your baby is probably close to sitting independently and laughing and squealing at anything remotely entertaining.

When to Introduce Solids

Watch for signs of readiness to take solids. The American Academy of Pediatrics recommends starting solids between four and six months of age. Compare this to what was being done in the 1950s when solids were introduced as early as a month or two of age. Many doting grandparents have asked me at the baby's two-month checkup if it is time to start solids . . . because their children had done fine on solids at that age. But there are medical reasons not to start solids too early. One concern has been that too many solids with their variety of proteins may trigger allergic reactions. This is especially true if there is a family history of allergies. Also, spooning food into the mouth of an infant who lacks the skills to show that he is no longer hungry may increase the likelihood that the child will learn to overeat.[56]

Following are some clues for readiness for solids. They do not all have to be present for you to begin offering solids.

- Your baby is watching you eat and opening his mouth or reaching for your food as you take a bite.

- He does not use his tongue to push objects out of his mouth.

- He is using a chewing motion with objects, not just the sucking motion.

- He has good head control and may be starting to sit by leaning forward on the arms for a few seconds.

- He is reaching and grabbing for objects and starting to move them toward the mouth.

- He is nursing more than 8 or 10 times a day and is not always satisfied after the feedings.

- If bottle feeding, he is taking more than 32 to 40 ounces a day in formula and may seem to want more.

- His birth weight has doubled.

Solid Sleep?

Many parents ask if their baby will sleep through the night if they start solids. Research seems to show that adding solids does not create a sleeping baby. However, my experience tells me that sometimes it does. If there has been a change in sleep and eating patterns where the baby seems hungrier and is eating more at night, solids in the evening may help.

Which Solids to Introduce

Cereal First

Let's say you've noticed your baby giving you the signals, and you are ready to start this new adventure. Most pediatricians recommend starting with rice cereal. It is bland and unlikely to cause any allergic reactions. It provides extra iron at a time when your baby needs more because the natural iron stores are depleted around six months of age. Start with a tablespoon of the dry rice cereal and mix it with breast milk or formula. Make it a loose consistency, like the consistency of applesauce. Use a rubber-tipped spoon for feeding. Stick with the rice cereal for a few weeks. It is not recommended to introduce rice cereal by putting it in a bottle of formula or breast milk or by using one of the infant feeders. Your baby will not learn the mechanics of eating solids, and there is a risk of feeding your baby unnecessary extra calories. The one exception is the baby who spits up excessively. (See p. 78, "Spitting Up.")

The attitude babies have with their first solids will vary. Some babies act like they have been eating solids all their life and are anxious for more. Some babies will make a face and tongue-thrust the food back out. It is probably not because your baby doesn't like it, but because he hasn't figured out what to do with it, or he is reacting to the new taste and texture. He needs to learn how to throw the food into the back of the mouth and then swallow.

What next?

After three or four weeks on the rice cereal or by six months of age, whichever comes first, you can start single-ingredient jarred foods. It may be helpful to try the vegetables first, because babies are born with that "sweet tooth." Try one new food every few days or even slower if there is a strong family history of allergies. Before six months of age, one or two varieties of fruit or vegetables may be introduced. In the next chapter we will talk about expanding the solids option.

Commercial (Conventional or Organic) Vs. Homemade

As far as the brand of solids to introduce (or whether to make your own), this is best based on your personal philosophy, your time allowances, and your budget. Obviously, ready-made foods are convenient and quick. Homemade foods will be more nutritious than ready-made foods. More variety can be offered with homemade foods. (See p. 92, "Homemade Foods.") When choosing commercial ready-to-eat baby food, you may decide to go with the conventional top brands *(Gerber, Heinz, and Beech-Nut)* or to choose an organic baby food brand *(Earth's Best, Well-Fed Baby, Gerber's Tender Harvest)*. Preservatives, artificial colors and flavorings, nitrates, and MSG are no longer found in baby foods. Read the label for ingredients such as sugar or modified food starch. These are not necessary and they may take the place of more nutritious ingredients.

Sixteen pesticides were found in trace amounts in eight different baby foods from *Gerber, Heinz,* and *Beech-Nut* in a 1997 report from the Environmental Working Group.[57] The amounts detected were well below safety standards, and these companies emphasize that they take precautions to reduce pesticides. The processing used in baby foods also helps to remove some of the pesticide residues. Environmental groups are calling for a separate set of pesticide standards for infants and young children, and concerns about the cumulative effect of pesticide exposure throughout the life of a child are being raised. With this in mind, how will you choose? Choosing to use more organic than conventionally grown foods may make sense due to the increased environmental exposure to toxins over a lifetime.

Great Eating Tips
for Babies
Four to Six Months

- **Sandwich the solids.** When starting out with solids, it is easiest to give your baby half the bottle of formula or half the usual nursing time, and then give the solids. After, the nursing or bottle can be finished. This way, your baby is not so hungry or so full that he is not able to focus on learning this new skill. If your baby has a tough time stopping the bottle or nursing halfway, then start with the solids and finish with the bottle or breast.

- **Pick your moments and relax.** Give solids when you are relaxed and not in a hurry. Babies need time to explore this new skill and need to feed at their own pace. In the beginning, if taking the time to feed solids does not fit into your schedule that day, you shouldn't worry about your baby missing solids here or there because he or she is still getting the majority of nutrition from formula or breast milk. Use small bites and allow your baby to finish each bite before starting the next one. Your baby needs to develop a sense of trust with you about feeding at this stage and if you are rushing through every bite, tension and frustration will appear.

- **Stop when the baby signals "stop."** Signals like turning the head or refusing to open the mouth mean "Enough!" There is no reason to force a certain amount of solids into your baby. Some days he may have a lot of interest in solids, and other days he may have no interest in them.

- **Try it, you'll like it!** A puckered-up face does not necessarily mean your baby doesn't like the food, but it may be a reaction to a new taste. Offer another spoonful if he is willing. If not, and he continues to refuse the food, don't get discouraged. Try again another day—you may get a different reaction. Try mixing it later with other foods that he does like. The tongue thrust that the baby still has may force a lot of the food right back out, but you can keep trying if he acts like he wants more.

- **Water, no juices.** Water may be introduced in a bottle or a cup. This may be especially important on hot days. Juices are not necessary at this age, and they may encourage your baby to prefer sweet fluids instead of water. (See p. 102, "What's the Problem with Juice?")

- **Stick with fruits and vegetables.** In this age group, rice cereal and maybe one or two varieties of fruits and vegetables may be tried. There is no reason to introduce meats or desserts.

- **Allow exploration with busy hands.** Babies love to dip their hands in the food and lick it off. Allow them freedom to explore.

- **Don't feed directly from the jar.** Transfer food from the jar to a bowl and feed. Leftover jars of food will be contaminated with your baby's saliva. The enzymes from the saliva will cause a breakdown of starch, and the bacteria from the saliva will multiply in leftover jars of food.

Chapter Five

roundup

Babies: Four to Six Months

- Formula intake should be around 25-32 ounces.

- Infants at this age need about 50 calories per pound of weight. Breast milk and formula are about 20 calories per ounce.

- Look for signs of readiness: your baby may watch you eat and open his mouth, be willing to chew objects and not thrust things back out with his tongue, and have good head control.

- Start with rice cereal for a few weeks.

- Add a fruit or vegetable if the rice cereal has been tolerated for 3 to 4 weeks.

- Introduce 1 new food every 3 or 4 days. Take more days if there is a family history of allergies.

- Start a cup around 5 to 6 months. Use water to start.

- Do not force or coax your baby to eat. If your baby is not interested, try another time.

- Allow the baby to explore solids with his fingers and hands (it's nothing a bath won't fix).

- Do not worry if some days your baby is not as interested or simply refuses the solids; the primary source of nutrition still comes from formula or breast milk.

- Solid intake will vary. Once to twice a day is sufficient. Once the baby is doing well with solids, $\frac{1}{4}$ to $\frac{1}{2}$ jar of food is average at one sitting.

Remember to relax, smile, be silly, laugh, sing, and enjoy!!

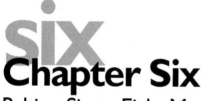

Chapter Six
Babies: Six to Eight Months

At six months of age, babies are very aware of their environment and want to interact with everything. They smile a lot, but can start to exhibit some of that "stranger anxiety." Sitting up and seeing the world of wonder is a favorite occupation of six-month-old babies. They are about to emerge into the world of mobility. How they choose to be mobile varies—rolling, scooting, squirming, crawling, and walking along furniture are all acceptable ways to be mobile at this age. The rate at which they choose to progress into mobility varies.

This age group is advancing in eating skill, and, of course, they want to be more involved, too. They will be taking more solids and will decrease their formula or breast milk intake accordingly. This is the time to introduce more varieties of foods. Don't get into a rut by offering the same foods over and over again. A variety of flavors may allow your baby to be more adventurous and open up those taste buds to new tastes later on. Don't be surprised, though, if your baby does start to develop some likes and dislikes. Some babies seem to be born with very discriminating palates.

What Kinds of Solids Now?

Cereals

Rice cereal is still a good choice, although you may move on to the infant oatmeal or barley cereals at this stage. It is better to use the dry cereals than the mixed jarred cereals. Eventually your baby should be taking about ½ cup a day of fortified baby cereal. The iron in the rice cereal helps to prevent iron deficiency anemia, the most common nutritional deficiency in children. A blood test for anemia is usually performed in the doctor's office sometime between 9 and 12 months of age. Cereals with wheat may be introduced after 7 or 9 months, but if there is a strong family history of food allergies, wait longer and watch for symptoms of food allergy. (See p. 74, "Facts on Food Allergies.")

Vegetables

Some babies may demonstrate their picky eating patterns by refusing certain types of vegetables. Consider combining some of the foods that they dislike with vegetables they do like or with rice cereal. Try not to combine them with the sweet fruits. The sweetness tends to overpower the flavor. If all they like are sweetened foods, where does this lead them later in their feeding experience? Try foods they refuse in a few weeks. They may have changed their mind. Encourage both green and yellow-orange vegetables.

Too much of the orange and yellow vegetables (like carrots, squash, and sweet potatoes) can cause a condition called *carotenemia*. This is where the baby's skin turns a yellow-orange color. This is not the same as the medical condition called *jaundice* that indicates a liver problem. With jaundice, the whites of eyes and body are yellow, but with carotenemia, the whites of the eyes stay white. Carotenemia is not a dangerous condition, but you are likely to get a lot of comments about your baby's suntan. By cutting down on the orange and yellow vegetables, the carotenemia will resolve. There may be a rare medical condition with carotenemia, but such children will not grow well and may have other problems such as vomiting or seizures.

Fruits

Many choices of jarred baby fruits are available. A consideration that may lead to choosing one fruit over another is whether your baby is constipated or having diarrhea.

- Constipating fruits: bananas and applesauce (cereals are also constipating)

- Loosening fruits: prunes, plums, pears, and peaches

Fresh fruits are more nutritious than the jarred variety. Preparing fresh fruits at home is easy.

Meats

Meats are rich in iron and protein, but high in fat. Historically, meats have been considered an essential part of a healthy diet, but recent research raises some concerns about the safety of meat for humans. The image of meat as a healthy part of our diet is changing, as discussed in Chapter 2. One question to consider is if babies need meats. Jarred baby meats and many of the mixed dinners have more fillers and many infants do not like the taste (maybe they are telling us something!). Some parents prefer to wait until their child can take finger food meats, and thus, avoid the processed baby food meats all together. There is no problem with doing this. Iron is being provided by breast milk, formula, and cereal, so babies are not missing iron if they are not fed meat.

Microwaving

When microwaving solids, make sure you use a microwave-safe dish. The food needs to only be lukewarm. Stir thoroughly to avoid "hot spots" and then test the temperature on your tongue or the back of your hand.

Homemade Foods

Making your own baby foods is a wonderful luxury and cheaper than buying baby foods. It really does not take that much extra time and by planning ahead and storing foods, it can become an easy routine. *Super Baby Food,* by Ruth Yaron, is an excellent resource for parents interested in homemade baby foods. Keep the following tips in mind when preparing homemade baby food.

- A small food processor, blender, or baby food grinder is a handy kitchen gadget to purée the foods.

- Use fresh fruits and vegetables in season. Certified organic produce is best and worth the extra cost when available. (See Chapter 2 and check out the resources in Appendix VI for organic food stores.) Canned fruits in natural juice, canned vegetables, or frozen varieties are also convenient. Avoid added salt, sugar, and butter in canned or frozen foods.

- Try to use fruits and vegetables within a day or two after you buy them. Vitamin C and the B vitamins are lost as the produce is stored. Wash and peel all fruits and vegetables.

- Fruits should be cooked for babies under 6 months of age. Bananas and avocados can be served mashed and raw for babies under 6 months of age. At 8 months you can start feeding soft fruits to your baby ripened, raw, and mashed. Fruits like melons, peaches, apricots, plums, mangoes, papayas, kiwis, and nectarines can be mashed and blended with some water to obtain a loose consistency.

- Firm fruits like apples and pears can be cooked in a small amount of water and then puréed for babies under 6 to 8 months of age.

- Steaming fruits and vegetables will help retain more nutrients. Save the cooking water from fruits or vegetables. It has a lot of the nutrients and can be added to thin out your purées.

- Avocados can be mashed and mixed with other foods or served alone. They are a great source of the "good fats" (and by the way, they are considered a fruit).

- Add a little lemon juice to fruit purée or avocado if you are not going to use it right away to prevent discoloration.

- Fresh vegetables that are easy to prepare and have low nitrate content include broccoli, potatoes, peas, and yams. (See box on High Nitrate Vegetables.) These may be cooked and puréed. Cook and purée the tender parts of the broccoli, cauliflower, and asparagus.

- To preserve nutrients while boiling fruits and vegetables, use very little water when you cook them. Cook until they are very soft, purée, and use only enough of the cooking water to loosen the consistency.

High Nitrate Vegetables

Certain areas of the country have more nitrates in the soil, especially if the soil is chemically over-fertilized. This has raised concerns about the presence of nitrates in certain vegetables, like beets, carrots, collard greens, spinach, and turnips. Because of a small risk of methemoglobinemia, (see p. 33, "Nitrates"), homemade varieties of these foods should not be fed to babies under about eight months of age. For these types of foods, commercial jarred baby foods may be safer for babies under eight months because the manufacturers test for nitrate contamination.

- Once you see your baby has done well on several fruits and vegetables, you may combine a few fruits or cook a few vegetables together and then blend.

- Add grains like brown rice, barley, oats, amaranth, millet, and quinoa to foods. Cook grains according to directions, purée, and add liquid to get a smooth consistency. (See p. 109, "The Goods on Grains.")

- Use tofu to mix with foods. It is a great protein source and can be introduced after eight or nine months of age.

- Use prepared baby foods that are stored in the refrigerator within a couple of days. Freeze small batches of your homemade fruits and vegetables in ice cube trays, transfer the frozen cubes to a freezer bag, and label and date. They can be stored for about two months in the freezer. They may be defrosted by leaving the needed portions covered in the refrigerator overnight or warming in the microwave or stovetop.

- There is no reason to add sugar, salt, or fats like butter to homemade baby foods.

- Herbs that are not spicy may be added in small amounts for flavor.

- To avoid choking risks, make sure the foods are smooth. Avoid stringy and chunky foods.

Self-Feeding Foods

Babies this age love to try to do everything by themselves. This is particularly true about eating. Babies will have their hands in the baby food, luxuriously lick it off, and then manage to get it all over their bodies as well. (Take some nice photos!) Babies at six to eight months will try to grab the spoon away from you and want to feed themselves. You can give your baby a second spoon to keep him distracted. Allow for the mess. It's an important part of the feeding process. He is ready for small, soft, cut-up finger foods when he develops that pincer grasp between the thumb and forefinger. He can try some thicker foods that he can get on his hands. Mounds of mashed potatoes or a small sticky rice ball with puréed food mixed in can be a way to start your baby with the skills of self-feeding. Some babies can handle small tastes of table food that are very soft. Teething biscuits, baby cookies, and baby crackers are tempting treats, but most contain sugar and hydrogenated oils. For example, the first few ingredients in Zwieback toast are enriched bleached flour, high fructose corn syrup, partially hydrogenated vegetable shortening (soybean oil), and sugar. There are some healthier varieties of baby crackers (e.g., *Earth's Best* and *Healthy Times*) at the health food store without the hydrogenated oils. These foods turn to mush in the mouth, but occasionally a baby will try for too big a bite and choke. Always supervise your baby while he is eating!

Foods to Avoid

Some foods can present health risks and some foods are not necessary for the young infant. Here is a list of some foods to avoid:

- Eggs until after a year of age: egg whites are allergenic for many infants.
- Products with nuts—another allergenic food.
- Some pediatricians recommend waiting before serving wheat and corn until after the baby is eight or nine months old; longer if there is a history of allergies.
- Honey until after a year of age. There is a risk of infant botulism from honey contaminated with the spores of *Clostridium botulinum.*
- Ready-made foods with added sugar or modified cornstarch.
- Ready-made baby foods like gelatin, pudding, and meat sticks, which have more fillers.
- Foods with trans fatty acids. These are the "bad fats" and in infants they have the potential to inhibit the use of the essential fatty acids, the "good fats" that are necessary for brain development.
- Citrus and tomatoes should be used cautiously under a year of age. They may cause rashes in the diaper area or around the mouth because of their acidity.
- Any hard, small pieces of foods that could be a choking hazard. (See p. 108, "Facts on Choking Hazards.")

Milk and Other Fluids

Babies should continue on breast milk or formula. As solid intake increases, the amount of milk will decrease. Twenty-four ounces is about the average daily intake. Juice is not necessary. (See p. 102, "What's the Problem with Juice?") Switch off between offering water and the formula or breast milk in the cup. This is so your baby will realize that formula and breast milk can come from a cup and not just from a bottle. When weaning off the bottle, some babies associate the milk with the bottle. They will than refuse to take the milk from the cup.

Great Eating Tips
for Babies
Six to Eight Months

- **Allow for messes.** Your baby will want to explore and use his hands to help you. Allow him to pick up food, even though it is bound to be a mess! If your baby is constantly grabbing your spoon to try to eat, give him an extra spoon to use. He may not accomplish much, but he'll have fun trying. He may be distracted enough to allow you to feed him. Parents who expect neatness are bound to create tension. Put a big sheet, mat, or newspapers under the high chair. Watch how you react to messes. If your baby is being messy and you are constantly interrupting the feeding rhythm by cleaning up or you are upset every time something spills, feeding will turn into a negative experience.

- **Work up to three times a day with solids.** Babies at this age should be able to get a breakfast, lunch, and dinner pattern with their solids. Don't worry about what you feed at each meal. Combinations of baby cereal, fruits, and vegetables are your best bet. Try to feed about $1/2$ cup of cereal (8 tablespoons of dry cereal) a day to ensure adequate iron intake.

- **Expect decreased formula/breast milk intake.** After six months of age, your baby should start to take two to three meals a day. Milk intake (still formula or breast milk) may diminish to around 20 to 25 ounces per day. If your baby is still taking over 32 ounces a day and full solids, discuss your baby's diet with your pediatrician to make sure the baby is not feeding too much.

• **Refusing solids?** Occasionally there is a baby in this age group who just doesn't seem that interested in the puréed solids. Make sure the baby is not so full with formula or breast milk before trying the solids. Be patient and don't panic! Babies vary developmentally and some just seem to have less interest. The other problem I see is that some just don't really enjoy this puréed stage and being spoon-fed. When the time comes for finger foods, their interest in food rises. However, I do encourage parents to keep trying. If you delay solid foods past seven or eight months, your baby may refuse textured foods when you finally do offer them.

• **Teething.** Very commonly, babies who are teething will show less interest in solids. Cool teething rings can be helpful for teething pain.

Please see the next section as many of the feeding issues of the six to eight-month old will have similar guidelines as the eight to twelve-month old. (See p. 103, "Great Eating Tips for Babies Eight to Twelve Months.")

Chapter Six
roundup
Babies: Six to Eight Months

- Formula or breast milk intake (about four nursings daily) is usually around 24 to 30 ounces per day. Babies at this age still need about 50 calories per pound of weight, however, more calories are starting to come from solids.

- Offer a variety of jarred or homemade puréed vegetables and fruits.

- If you choose to make your own foods, avoid adding sugar, salt, or butter.

- Limit or consider holding off on meats until later.

- Work up to offering meals with solids three times a day.

- Use smooth baby foods.

- Offer a cup.

- Give your baby a spoon to play with while feeding.

- Allow your baby to decide how much to eat.

- Avoid commercial fruit juices.

seven
Chapter Seven
Babies: Eight to Twelve Months

Action begins here! Getting into things they shouldn't be getting into is this age group's most desired activity. Remote controls, telephones, electric cords, computer keyboards, cabinets, and paper are the most desired objects. Forget all the expensive toys that the grandparents bought—the parents' toys are much more exciting. Mobility is being mastered at this age. It is hard to keep up with, much less catch, this high-speed crawling machine. Then watch out—they're off and running!

This stage offers the transition to feeding finger or table foods and independent eating. The transition through this stage may progress very fast or more slowly. Again, we must let our infant set the pace, but we must be ready to hold tight and continue offering lots of healthy choices. It seems so tempting to allow our baby to snack constantly on those little fish-shaped crackers to give us peace in the car or while waiting for an appointment, but avoid this trap! You'll pay the price later.

If we rushed our baby into walking or restrained him from trying because it would be easier to carry him, how would he achieve this amazing milestone? Similarly, feeding is a time where a parent must exhibit both patience and restraint. We must be patient in allowing our baby to develop the skills to self-feed and not rush our baby. We must show restraint in not taking over the feedings completely because it is easier, faster, or less messy.

When to Introduce Finger Foods

Developmentally, watch for the pincer grasp. This is when an infant is able to grab small objects between the thumb and forefinger. Infants between eight and ten months also start to develop more of a chewing motion. When this occurs, the child is ready to handle finger foods. Babies don't need teeth to start with soft finger foods (some don't get their first tooth until after a year of age). Try putting a few pieces of finger foods cut up in small bite-size pieces on the tray table. While he or she is eating the finger foods, you can still slip in the puréed jarred foods with the spoon. The finger foods offer a bit of independent distraction for the busy infant who is trying to explore and put everything in the mouth. Gradually he or she will get better at handling the finger foods and will do less with baby foods. Some babies quickly discover the wonders of finger foods and refuse the puréed stuff as they get more proficient with self-feeding.

The Baby Who Gags on Food

Beware of "gaggers." These are babies who have trouble handling any type of chunky food or finger foods because they gag and choke. Some babies are going to be slower to progress to finger foods because of this problem. Some babies have difficulty with the stage-three type foods, which are puréed with chunks. They are not sure whether to let it slip down like a smooth food or chew it up like a finger food, so they gag. Don't fret; I've never known a five-year-old who has to eat baby food. All babies will eventually move onto table and finger foods. However, with some it may be after a year of age. Don't be alarmed if your baby does gag occasionally. Some babies simply try to overstuff their mouths when they are eating, and this will lead to the gag. Offer appropriate, soft finger foods and not "chokable" types of finger foods. (See p. 108, "Facts on Choking Hazards.") Try not to overreact if your baby gags. Some babies will seek the attention (your reaction of screaming or grabbing him or her) and will purposely try to gag to get the attention. Stay calm, and if your child is making noise and gagging, the little one is unlikely to be in trouble. I strongly urge having a CPR course under your belt so you'll know what to do in case of an emergency. Also, be alert that babies with this wonderful new pincer grasp are now able to find all sorts of non-edible choking hazards around the house.

What Types of Finger Foods

Foods that are soft and cut into bite-size pieces are appropriate finger foods. Firmer foods can be offered if they dissolve easily in the mouth. Some babies try to shove everything that can fit into their mouths, therefore place only small quantities of food before them at a time. Fruits and vegetables should be the mainstays of the diet for this age group, although more grains and other protein sources can be introduced.

As far as spending the extra money for jarred diced fruits and vegetables, baby meat sticks, and even the third-stage foods—they are probably best left on the shelves of your grocery store. Save yourself some money; you are much better off dicing your own fruits and vegetables and finding healthier sources of protein that taste better. Mash up your own mixed dinners to create a healthy "third-stage type" dinner. Yours will be more nutritious, tastier, and your baby will love you for it.

Fruits

- Try bananas, mangoes, watermelon, cantaloupe, apricots, papayas, pears, peaches, plums, and nectarines.
- Use canned fruits in natural juices.
- Citrus fruits should be introduced closer to a year of age. Watch for rashes around the mouth and in the diaper area.
- Apples should be sliced thin and cut up.

Vegetables

- Vegetables should be steamed, boiled, baked, or microwaved until soft.
- Try cooked carrots, peas, broccoli tops, asparagus tips, avocados, squashes, zucchini, potatoes, and sweet potatoes. You don't need to worry about the nitrates in purchased produce after your baby is eight months old. Infants of this age are less likely to be affected.
- Frozen or canned vegetables can be used. Avoid those with added salt or butter. Frozen vegetables are more nutritious than the canned variety.

Dairy

- To avoid aspartame and sugar, plain yogurt can be mixed with puréed fruit. *Stonyfield* and *Horizon* make organic yogurt. Use whole milk or low-fat yogurt, because babies need the extra fat. If you buy the yogurt with fruit, watch for chunks of fruit. The mixture of "smooth" with "chunks" can be difficult for some babies to handle. Look for yogurt with "live and active cultures." These contain beneficial bacteria.
- Grated cheese and cottage cheese can be offered.
- Vegetarian soy cheese is also available.

Meat/Protein Group

- Soft chicken, turkey, and ground meats can be given although I tell parents they are not necessary. Some babies have a harder time with meats until after a year of age. Meats boiled and softened in soups can be easier for them to handle. (See p. 30, "Hormones and Antibiotics in Meat.")
- Try tofu as an alternative protein source. Add to yogurt, pasta, and rice dishes.
- Beans and legumes will need to be mashed or puréed. They can be added to rice, pasta dishes, or mixed with vegetables.
- Try vegetarian burgers (like *Gardenburgers*) broken up in small pieces.
- Avoid fish because of the mercury issue. (See p. 31, "Mercury.")

Grains

- Offer rice, pasta, bread, oatmeal, dry cereal, pancakes, or waffles (no need for syrup or butter).

- You can find more creative types of pasta, primarily found in health food stores. Made from amaranth, quinoa, and even from lentils, these will add some variety and are an easy way to increase whole grains.

- Make balls of mashed potatoes or rice, and add other finger foods to them for an edible food ball.

- Add mashed avocado to cooked pasta. Instead of the classic "mac and cheese" from a box, make your own pasta and add cottage cheese or your own grated cheese or soy cheese.

- Try bread, bread sticks, and crackers. Supervise to make sure the baby doesn't try to bite off too big a chunk. Try to find the brands of crackers and baby cookies without hydrogenated oils in the health food store. *Earth's Best* makes teething biscuits without the hydrogenated oils. If you have concerns about allergies, wait on the wheat products until after the baby's first year.

- Experiment with other grains like amaranth, quinoa, couscous—add to other foods for texture. (See p. 109, "The Goods on Grains.")

Foods to Use Sparingly

- Dried fruits are sticky and can promote tooth decay. If you do buy dried fruit, purchase dried fruit without the sulfites, a food preservative. Sulfites can trigger asthma attacks in about 5 to 10 percent of asthma sufferers.

Foods to Avoid

- Processed foods like lunch meats with nitrates and foods with colorings and preservatives. (See p. 33, "Nitrates.")

- Sugary cereals. (See p. 110 to see how to choose healthier cereals.)

- Eggs until after a year of age because of the risk of an egg allergy.

- Honey until after a year of age because of the risk of botulism.

- Condiments like catsup (which is 29 percent sugar) and soy sauce (high in salt) are not necessary.

- Candy, chocolate, cookies, and cakes do not need to be a part of the infant diet.

- Hot dogs and grapes are choking hazards.

Milk and Other Fluids

Continue letting your baby practice with the cup. Formula or breast milk should still be used until a year of age and should be offered in the cup on occasion. Give water in a cup, too. Start using a combination of the "sippy"cup with a lid and an open cup. The open cups are messier, but babies should practice this skill with a small amount of fluid. Juices are not necessary. An occasional serving of fruit or vegetable juices or homemade juices can be used. See the box below for the scoop on juice.

What's the Problem with Juice?

- Juice can cause diarrhea in many children. Juice contains a large amount of sugar, like fructose and sorbitol, that may lead to diarrhea, often called "toddler's diarrhea." Sorbitol is present in prune juice and apple juice, but not in white grape juice or orange juice. The high amounts found in prune juice are what give it its laxative effect. Drinking too much sorbitol-containing juice can cause a child to suffer cramps, gas, and diarrhea.

- Juice can lead to tooth decay, especially for older infants. If babies have a constant juice bottle, the sugar is constantly coating the teeth. Never give your baby a juice bottle before naps or bedtime.

- Juice fills children up so they may not be hungry for more nutritious foods. When juice is offered with a meal or right before a meal, the sugar suppresses the appetite. Drinking the sweet stuff now may set them up for craving sodas later on.

- Juice does not have high nutritional value. Although juice is fortified with vitamins, food is actually a better source of vitamins and fiber than juice.

- The American Academy of Pediatrics (AAP) policy on juice states that children between 1 and 6 years should drink no more than 6 ounces of juice a day; children 7 years and older should drink less than 12 ounces of juice a day.

- The AAP states that juice should not be given before 6 months of age. In my own practice, I encourage parents to wait until after the baby is a year old. It is better to have the child be used to water and not the sweet drinks when you are ready to wean from the bottle to a cup after a year. Diluting juices helps control the overdrinking of juice.

Daycare and Other Caretakers

A child who is in daycare or with a baby sitter all day may learn different signals for eating. It is important that you review eating habits with your providers so that you understand their approach to feeding. Questions to consider asking your daycare provider or sitter might include:

- What type of foods and snacks are being offered? Are fruits and vegetables offered regularly? Do parents have any influence over what is served at daycare?

- When are snacks offered? Are they offered at a regular time, available all the time, or distributed on request?

- What fluids are offered and when? Is juice, water, or milk available at mealtime, snacks, or whenever the child wants? Will they provide you with a menu?

- How do they handle the picky eater? Do they continue to offer choices?

- Are junk food, candy, and sweets around often or easily available?

- Are safety issues addressed such as non-chokable food choices?

If you have a caretaker in your home, you will have more control over food choices based on what you buy and have available in the house. If your child is in daycare, you should try to make sure the provider's methods of feeding do not conflict with your basic principles.

Great Eating Tips
for Babies
Eight to Twelve Months

- **Cup, cup, cup.** Make a habit of offering a cup. The lidded "sippy" cup will save you clean-up time after the spills. As your baby's coordination improves, offer the cup without a lid for practice. Bottle weaning should occur by 12 to 15 months. Use water, but also try using formula or breast milk in the cup to help with bottle weaning.

- **Variety, variety, variety.** Offer a variety of tastes and flavors. Let your baby try lots of new foods. Don't get into a rut. Experiment with new fruits and vegetables yourself. Focus on fruits and vegetables as the main part of the meals. At six months, start with the single-ingredient fruits and vegetables, and then move into the combination foods. Watch for the pincer grasp as a sign to start soft finger foods. Initially, offer some of these finger foods to allow your baby to practice. He or she will gradually improve these skills and will eventually prefer finger foods over puréed foods. Then it is time to move into the variety of finger foods.

- **Avoid desserts.** Use fruit as dessert. Jarred desserts and puddings have added sugar and little nutritional value.

- **Schedules and sitting for meals.** Babies should develop a three-meal-a-day routine plus one or two snacks a day by the end of the first year. However, the infant less than a year old is making the transition into this pattern, so some days may vary. Sometimes it is hard to expect babies to wait until the family is together to eat dinner. It may be easier to feed your baby his main meal ahead of time and then have him sit during the family mealtime with a cup or a few finger foods. This helps to develop the socialization at mealtime that is important later on. Don't start the habit of using constant snacks to keep your baby distracted.

- **Allow your baby to set the pace.** Some babies can't get the food in their mouths fast enough. Some babies dawdle and are easily distracted. Keep up with your baby's tempo for feeding. Some are more adventurous and will try everything in sight, while others are picky and reject certain flavors or textures. Accept and enjoy the way your baby approaches food. If you are irritated by his or her approach to food, this will make feeding a negative experience.

- **Minimize outside distractions.** Turn off the television while your baby is eating. Other kids playing may also create a distraction so that your baby may be less interested in eating.

- **Allow your baby to regulate the amount of food.** As tempting as it is to have your baby finish what you are serving, allow him or her to decide how much to eat. Expect a variation in appetite from meal to meal and from day to day. How many of us are convinced we know how much our child should be eating? When the baby takes two bites and shows all signs of being finished, the parent tries to coax and force the baby into taking more bites. Remember that you can choose what to offer your child, but you can't choose how much food he will eat. Trust your baby's appetite, even if your instincts disagree.

- **Stick to your choices.** If your baby is refusing the two or three choices you are offering, don't be tempted to bring out a smorgasbord of other choices, especially if they are less healthy ones. I knew one mother who realized her daughter would always eat those fish-shaped crackers. If her baby refused a meal, she would offer her crackers. By one year of age, that was the main staple of the child's diet. The baby had figured out that by refusing food, she would always get what she really wanted.

- **Babies who throw and drop food.** Why do all babies insist on doing this? They have discovered the law of gravity. It is fun to drop things and watch them disappear. It is also a time for them to learn about "object permanence," that is, that the object still exists even when it is out of sight. Don't get upset. Sometimes, they see that they get a reaction and it becomes a game for them. If they only throw an occasional morsel of food, ignore it. If they seem to be finished eating and decide that throwing their food or plate off the tray table is their signal they are done, calmly pick up the plate and declare that mealtime is over. There are many great products on the market now like a baby bowl with a suction cup on the bottom so the bowl stays put. It may be worth the investment.

- **Illnesses.** When your baby is sick, expect a decrease in appetite and, at times, a complete refusal of solid foods. This is fine as long as your baby is drinking well and staying hydrated.

Check out Dr. Wood's *Call Your Pediatrician* Web site to find out the signs of dehydration and what to do when your child is sick. **www.callyourped.com**

- **Safety tips.** Never leave your baby unattended during mealtime. Watch for older children offering inappropriate foods to the baby. If your baby is sitting in your lap to feed, do not have hot liquids around that could be knocked over and cause a burn. Avoid hard foods that are choking hazards. (See p. 108, "Facts on Choking Hazards.") If your baby is starting to eat finger foods, make sure they are soft or will dissolve easily.

Chapter Seven

roundup

Babies: Eight to Twelve Months

- Allow for the new independence your baby will be experiencing in self-feeding.

- Formula or breast milk intake should be around 20 to 25 ounces a day.

- Watch for the pincer grasp and offer soft, bite-size foods. You can still spoon-feed puréed foods in between bites.

- Offer a cup with water, formula, or breast milk. Avoid commercial juices.

- Introduce a variety of foods and flavors. Primarily use fruits and vegetables, and try to limit processed foods like crackers and cookies.

- Limit choices to two or three at mealtime, and don't be tempted to offer several choices at every meal because your baby refuses your initial offerings.

- Minimize your reaction to your baby's dropping food.

- Discuss feeding practices with your daycare provider or sitter.

- Don't use food as a distraction or a way to keep your baby occupied.

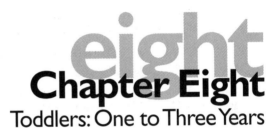

Chapter Eight
Toddlers: One to Three Years

The Great Birthday has arrived: ONE! It seems that once a baby hits age one, everything changes. Activity and endless energy are the names of the game for toddlers. Because most have accomplished the feat of walking, they are burning up more energy than ever: therefore most toddlers start to lose their baby fat. The cuddly dependent baby you have grown accustomed to in the first year is changing into an opinionated, independent, curious toddler. (Some parents tell me it happens overnight.)

Toddlers challenge limits. Feeding, which used to be a necessary and focused activity, can change into a chaotic, limit-testing battleground. Some days as a parent you may want to tear your hair out, and other days you find yourself laughing at new behaviors. Toddlers do need limits, and as parents, this is the most difficult part of parenting a toddler. How far do you go in setting limits and how do you set them? There are entire books on this subject, but if you are having difficulty feeding your toddler AND other behaviors are out of control, you may need to examine your discipline techniques.

Discuss your concerns with your pediatrician. This is the age to address these issues because toddlers who are not handled well can turn into difficult preschoolers, elementary school age children, and then teens.

Feeding toddlers has its special challenges. Toddlers have so many other new skills they are learning that feeding is no longer a priority in their life. Eating creates lots of new opportunities for your toddler to test limits. Parents tend to worry about the diminished appetite that occurs at this age. **A decrease in appetite in this age group is normal.** A toddler's weight gain will slow down during this period, and thank goodness, for if they continued to grow at the rate of the first year of life, you would have a 40- to 50-pounder by age two! Toddlers only gain about 3 to 5 pounds a year. At the 15- or 18-month checkup, many parents seem crestfallen that the weight gain has been so little, but this is normal! There is a natural decline in toddlers' appetites that is hard for some parents to deal with, but it is a natural process.

Pick Your Battles

Research shows that children are capable of regulating their intake according to their energy needs. It also shows that children of parents who were the most controlling about food were the least able to adjust and compensate their caloric intake. You are in control of what you buy and offer your toddler. If you beg, threaten, bribe, or force your toddler into eating, you will be the loser. Studies show that they will actually eat less, so this is not a battle you want to fight!

Healthy Food Ideas for Toddlers

One important rule is to avoid hard, chokable foods. Most choking incidents occur when a child is running around or laughing or playing while eating. As they progress through the one-to three-year stage, they will gradually be able to handle more hard foods.

Facts on Choking Hazards

- Most children who choke on food are under three years of age.

- Two-thirds of the foods aspirated are inappropriate foods for infants and toddlers. One-fourth of the foods are fruits and vegetables.

- Unsafe foods include nuts, popcorn, seeds (e.g., pumpkin or sunflower seeds), Corn Nuts, hard candy, jelly beans, hot dogs (unless cut lengthwise in quarters), chunks of peanut butter, raw carrots or celery, grapes (unless cut in quarters), large chunks of meat, or hard fruits.

- Children under four years of age should be taught to eat only while sitting down and to not overstuff their mouths with food.

- Never let toddlers eat unattended. Never allow them to eat while running and playing.

- Some experts advise that foods like hot dogs, hard pieces of fruit, and raw vegetables should not be given to children younger three.

• If your child has a coughing episode after choking on food and then develops wheezing, trouble breathing, or a persistent cough, seek immediate medical attention for a possible foreign body aspiration.

Grains

• Rice: Try adding bits of cut-up vegetables and small pieces of chicken, turkey, or fish to rice. If your toddler is the type to pick out things, buy an extra-fine grater for the vegetables, or purée and mix with the rice. Brown rice is more nutritious with more protein, fiber, zinc, folic acid, and vitamin E than white rice.

• Pasta: Try spinach, tomato, and wheat pastas for variety and color. Some newer varieties appearing on the shelves of health food stores are made from lentils, amaranth, and quinoa (see "The Goods on Grains" below). Rainbow pasta is a great way to teach colors by having your toddler eat all the green, then the red and yellow pastas. Chop up spinach, grate zucchini and carrots, and any other vegetables you can think of and add to the pasta and sauces.

The Goods on Grains

"Whole grains" are getting more attention these days. The most common grains people are familiar with are wheat, corn, oats, and rice. See "Facts on Wheat" (p. 110) to learn how to buy the healthiest parts of the wheat. Look for other grains in the health food store. Many stores have bins of raw grains where you can buy a small quantity. Experiment and find ways to cook them and add them to your family's diet. Other grains worthy of trying include:

Amaranth: A tiny seed packed with protein, iron, and calcium. It can be cooked in water or popped like popcorn in a pan with dry heat. It has a nutty flavor. The toasted seed can be added to cereal or baked goods. It can be cooked with other grains.

Barley: High in protein and fiber. Often used in soups. Pearled barley has the outer husk removed and cooks in less time, but has less nutritional value than barley.

Buckwheat: High in B vitamins, and good in pancakes, bread, and hot cereals.

Kamut: This is a bread grain with 40 percent more protein than wheat.

Millet: High in B vitamins, copper, and iron. Cooked millet can be cooled and formed into patties and refried for millet burgers. Found in breads in its raw form.

Oats: Most people are familiar with oats as a cereal or as an addition to granola, breads, muffins, or cookies.

Quinoa: The highest amount of protein of any grain. It cooks quickly and can be served in a pilaf, sauces, or cooked as a cereal.

- Whole wheat breads (see "Facts on Wheat" in the box below), rice cakes, pita breads: Pita bread can be baked and sprinkled with Parmesan cheese. If your child is constipated, look for high-fiber breads. There are some bran breads with up to 5 grams of fiber per slice.
- Healthy cereals: Check the labels. You can find healthier choices. Remember the study in the first chapter showed that the majority of children receive their vitamins and nutrients from cereal? Consider your choices carefully. Once you start down the path of sugar-filled cereal, it is hard to turn back. You can try mixing your child's less healthy varieties with more healthy varieties. Features to look for include:
    - Less than 6 grams of sugar per 1-ounce serving
    - No hydrogenated oils or chemical preservatives (BHA or BHT preservatives may cause allergic reactions or increase cancer risks)
    - Fiber content over 5 grams
    - Grains should be "whole wheat" or "wheat bran"
    - Protein content over 3 grams per serving

  You may not find all of these features in the cereal, but the more you can strive for, the better. The first two features are probably the most important.
- Pizza. Make healthy pizzas on pita bread or English muffins. Spread with tomato sauce. Make faces with cheese slices or string cheese smiles, olive eyes, and a bell pepper nose.

Facts on Wheat

- Breads that list "*whole wheat*" or "*100 percent whole wheat*" contains both the outer bran layer, which is rich in fiber, and the inner germ of the wheat kernel, which contains vitamin B-6, vitamin E, copper, folate, magnesium, and zinc.
- Breads that list "*wheat flour*" or "*wheat*" are refined from white flour (75 percent) and wheat flour (25 percent) and the bran and germ are not present. With the outer nutritional layer of the wheat seed stripped, over 20 nutrients and the fiber are diminished. Vitamins and minerals are then added

back and the bread is called "fortified." When you see the terms "enriched," "refined," or "bleached," these are processes that make the grain less nourishing.

- Always look for the word *"whole"* or *"multi-whole grain"* on the label to make sure you are getting the healthiest type of grains.

- Encourage your child to eat 100 percent whole wheat bread early on and avoid white bread.

Fruits and Vegetables

- Fruits are usually easy for toddlers to love because of their natural sweetness. Offer fresh varieties that are in season. If your child's favorite fruits are not available fresh, then purchase them canned in natural juices or buy frozen fruit. Another favorite is to make homemade popsicles with fruit. Purée fruits with a little water, fruit juice, or yogurt. Place the mixture in small paper cups with a popsicle stick, ice cube trays, or in store-bought popsicle makers and freeze. Grapes plucked off the stem can be frozen for a healthy treat. Offer fruits as snack options and as dessert.

- Vegetables can be more of a challenge. Always offer a few bites of vegetables with meals. Try a variety of vegetables (this may mean experimenting yourself with some new foods). When my son was three, we discovered he loved to eat artichokes and soybeans. He loved scraping the artichoke leaves with his teeth, and he loved squeezing the soybean out of the skin. It was the process of eating these foods that intrigued him. They were not what I would have thought as "kid-favorite foods," but he loved them. Remember to stay neutral about children eating their vegetables. When parents force the vegetables, toddlers will often refuse them. Raw vegetables are usually not tolerated until around three years of age. For the ultra-picky vegetable eater, here are some suggestions:

    - Finely grate vegetables and melt them in a cheese sandwich or quesadilla or add them to peanut butter, pasta, rice, soups, or macaroni and cheese.

    - Grate vegetables and add them to pancake batter, muffin batter, or scrambled eggs.

    - Add a slice of tomato, cucumber, cooked carrots, or vegetable juice to a fruited yogurt smoothie drink.

    - Sprinkle peas or corn on yogurt or frozen yogurt and call them "sprinkles."

Meat and Meat Alternatives

- Offer lean meats and use more chicken or turkey than red meat. Many toddlers will not eat red meat items like steak because it is too chewy.

- Limit hot dogs and processed lunch meat because of the nitrate content. (Remember that hot dogs can be a choking hazard and should be cut up.) Shelton's makes a hot dog without nitrates that can be found in the frozen section of some health food stores. (See p. 33, "Nitrates.")

- Use beans and lentils in soups and casseroles, or mash them and add to items like a rolled tortilla with cheese.

- Peanut butter should be smooth, not chunky. Spread a thin layer on a cracker or piece of bread.

- Serve fish without bones and try some of the oily varieties (rich in the omega-3 essential fatty acids) like mackerel, salmon, and herring. Farmed fish (like salmon) probably have less toxins in them. (See p. 31 "Mercury.")

Milk and Dairy Products

- Use whole milk until two years of age, after that switch to 2 percent or 1 percent. (See below, "Fats for Toddlers.")

- Calcium requirements at this age are 500 mg a day. This would be met by drinking 12 ounces of milk. The child should not be drinking more than about 20 to 24 ounces of milk per day. If he is, he may be filling up on milk and missing nutrition from other sources.

- If your child is allergic to milk, try rice milk or soy milk (but keep in mind that many children with a true milk allergy are also allergic to soy). Rice milk and soy milk can be found fortified with calcium, but they are low in fat and protein. In this age group, you must be careful of using these milks. I recommend using an omega-3 oil supplement regularly to provide the "good fats" that are important in brain development if a child in this age group needs to stay on these low-fat milks. (See p. 55, "Fats: The Good, the Bad, and the Ugly.") There have been reports of children receiving the majority of their nutrition from these drinks and then having problems with their growth and nutritional deficiencies (like protein deficiencies). There are also soy-based and rice-based ice creams.

Fats for Toddlers

- Make sure you are offering whole milk, not 2 percent, 1 percent, or non-fat milk until after 2 years of age. Toddlers need the extra fat for brain development. They may receive more than 40 percent of their daily calories as fat. This does not mean allowing unlimited fat and butter.

- Once children have reached 2 years of age, decrease milk to 1 percent or 2 percent. If you feel your toddler is overweight, talk to your pediatrician to see if this is really the case. Many toddlers appear chubby, but are proportional on the growth curves. If your toddler is on the heavy side, you may want to use 1 percent milk.

- The 1995 Dietary Guidelines Advisory Committee recommended that there be a gradual change in dietary fat intake between the ages of 2 and 5 towards the heart-healthy diet. The adult heart-healthy diet contains 30 percent of calories from fat, less than 10 percent of calories from saturated fat, and less than 300 milligrams per day of cholesterol. However, new studies show that limiting fat in children over age 2 to 30 to 35 percent fat of daily calories did not compromise brain development.[58]

- If children have lactose intolerance, they may have cramps, diarrhea, and gassiness after consuming milk products. This reaction is genetic and tends to be common in African, Asian, and Native American people. It usually appears at about age three or four. This is not an allergy, but these children do not have the enzyme in their intestinal tract to break down the lactose in milk. Your choices are to use rice, soy, reduced-lactose, or lactose-free milk (*Lactaid* is a popular brand). Alternatively, lactase enzyme, available over-the-counter, can be taken with milk products. It is available in drops that can be taken with the milk products.

- Yogurt can be plain with your own fresh fruit added or used as part of a smoothie shake. Try to avoid the gimmick yogurt with the sprinkles (it's just sugar). Also, avoid aspartame additives. Use your own healthy sprinkles at home like wheat germ, granola, cereal, crushed nuts, or toasted amaranth seeds. Remember that children this age can easily choke on whole nuts. Add tofu to the smoothie for a good serving of protein.

- Add fresh fruit to cottage cheese for a healthy breakfast or put it on bread or in a pita pocket.

Our Healthy Smoothie

1 cup of cold water

6 frozen strawberries or other frozen fruit

1 banana

1 scoop soy protein powder*

1 scoop fiber powder*

2 tsps. flaxseed oil*

*products from **USANA** (see Appendix VI)

Great Eating Tips
for Toddlers
Ages One to Three

- **Offer a wide variety of fresh foods.** The majority of the foods offered should be fruits, vegetables, and grains. Limit exposure to processed foods like crackers, cookies, candy, granola bars, chips, and fruit roll-ups. I'm not saying to give up these foods, but use fresh foods as snacks and pick healthier types of processed food snacks, like pretzels instead of potato chips. Use foods such as candy, cookies, and cake as rare treats, not as part of the daily diet. Your child will be exposed to these eventually (they're impossible to avoid). Repeated opportunities to try a new food will generally produce a liking for the new food, although five to ten exposures are often required.[59]

- **Have regular meals and snacks.** Snacks should be planned and constant snacking should be discouraged. If your toddler cruises around and is constantly grazing on handouts and snacks, he will not be hungry for his meal. Encourage eating fresh fruit as a snack. Avoid giving snacks while the child is watching television. This habit can lead to excess weight gain.

- **Make meals a family event.** For most families, this will occur primarily at dinner. The television should be off. The interaction should be pleasant, although we all know toddlers have their bad days (so do parents). Focus on the conversation and not the food. Don't talk about unpleasant topics or bring arguments to the dinner table. Even toddlers understand anger and stress and will be less likely to focus on eating.

- **Start to develop responsibility.** Allow the toddler some responsibility for mealtime, like putting the napkins out. Let him or her help with preparation when it is developmentally appropriate. Activities like drying lettuce with paper towels can be a big accomplishment for a toddler (the salad spinner is also a fun "toy"). Pouring an ingredient into a mixture can be a fun task for toddlers. Obviously, keep safety issues in mind around the kitchen.

- **Give choices.** Children cooperate more often when they get to choose (for example, which plate or cup they want or which of two vegetables they want at lunch). But don't overwhelm them with food choices—give them only one decision to make at a time.

- **Develop mealtime expectations for behavior.** A one-year-old is still expected to play with his food, but a three-year-old should be able to develop some mealtime manners. If your older toddler is being disruptive and displaying poor manners, he can be excused for a short period. If your toddler is not interested in the meal, you can see if he can just sit and keep you company for part of the meal. If his attention is lost, allow him to get down, but don't let him take handouts off the table and cruise around. Allow him to develop independent eating skills as he develops coordination. Continuing to try to spoon-feed a 1-year-old is bound to lead to some battles. Allow for the messes. At 15 to 20 months, he will begin to develop the capability to use utensils.

- **Food art and creativity.** Creative ways to present food can be a way to get kids to try new things. Shapes and colors are something they are learning at this age, so play games like "Simon says pick and eat a green food." Cut food into fun shapes or use them to make designs on the plate, like faces and animals. Use cheese slices and vegetable combinations to decorate a pita bread or an English muffin pizza. Add fruit slices, dried fruit, and yogurt hair to decorate pancakes. Fill ice cream cones with yogurt or cottage cheese and sprinkle with fruit. Get creative cookie cutters and cut up vegetables, like cucumbers, or parboiled carrots into shapes. Ask him to eat the different shapes. Serve a mystery food (like a new fruit or vegetable): put it in a paper bag and see who can feel and guess the food. Have the child put a hand in, grab the food, and take a bite without looking and guess the food. Play the blind bite game: the parent gets to place a bite of any food into the child's mouth with his eyes closed and the child has to guess which food it is. A funny song or saying that goes with a certain food can keep eating entertaining. You don't want to overdo it with all the games, but it can be an occasional way to make trying new things fun.

- **Serve your child the same foods that the family is eating.** If your toddler chooses not to eat what is served, do not allow him to get a second choice for a meal, or he will start to expect it. Don't be a short-order cook. Offer a variety of foods at meals: a main dish, a fruit or vegetable, bread or rice, and milk. Include one choice in the group that you know your toddler is likely to accept. Offer the foods in a neutral manner, not by pressuring him into eating more of one or the other. If he refuses to eat the main dish, he still has the side dishes of vegetables, rice, or bread. Don't go back to the kitchen to cook another meal.

- **"Can I have dessert?"** When kids ask about dessert, don't use the standard reply your parents and grandparents used, "If you eat all your dinner, THEN you can get dessert." This places a lot of value on dessert and less value on the meal itself. Never bribe with dessert. Treats like ice cream, cookies, and cake are fine for toddlers to have, but having them as a regular part of every meal is not a good habit to develop. Never giving sweets or treats may also be detrimental. When kids are older they may seek out foods they were deprived of. Try to limit temptation by buying only small quantities of treats and having periods where there are no desserts in the house. You can honestly say, "We don't have any cake or ice cream," and then you can offer fruit for dessert. Instead of keeping a big tub of ice cream in the freezer, have an occasional outing to the ice cream store. Use fruit as the most frequent dessert offered. It can be served with a small amount of ice cream, pudding, or yogurt. Does your child hold back on dinner, so he or she can fill up on dessert? Try this approach: serve a reasonable-sized portion of dessert with the meal. Of course, your child will choose to eat that first, but then what? He or she has "permission" now to eat dinner and since dessert is out of the way, there is no "saving themselves."

> **WARNING:** This may mean changing some of your own dessert habits, but these changes are likely to be positive changes for you! Do *you* really need to have rich desserts every night?

- **Offer small amounts of food.** Portions are small for toddlers. Guidelines for a serving size from the Food Guide Pyramid are about one to two tablespoons of vegetables per year of age, one-half ounce of meat, half a piece of fruit, half a slice of bread, half a cup of milk or half an ounce of cheese, and a quarter cup of cereal, rice, or pasta. By using small portions, you will allow your toddler to be more successful in eating and maybe even ask for seconds. Estimated caloric intake for a one to three-year-old is about 40 calories per inch of height.

- **Allow toddlers to follow their natural instincts for eating and fullness.** We have all heard "have two more bites" or "clean your plate." If children are full, allow them to recognize that signal. Not allowing that recognition may lead them to ignore those signals later in life, which could lead to obesity. Many toddlers eat well for breakfast or lunch and have very little at dinner. For parents whose focus is on the evening meal, this can be distressing. When my son was 18 months old, my daycare provider declared him the biggest eater in the daycare. It was hard for me to believe based on his dinner performance, but it did help to reassure me that he was capable of eating well. Appetites will vary from meal to meal and from day to day. Allow for this normal regulation. If you find that your child is a great breakfast or lunch eater, serve more variety at those meals. Fruits and vegetables for a toddler's breakfast are fine.

- **Fad foods and food strikes.** Sometimes toddlers will get stuck on one food that they seem to crave every day. There is no harm in this as long as it is a nourishing food. Always place other choices on the plate with the fad food. A week later, toddlers are likely to declare that they hate the same food they demanded the previous week. Refusing to eat at all is another toddler issue. Don't show your anxiety or concern. Sometimes, if you ignore the issue, toddlers will start eating once they see that the family is eating. If they continue to refuse to eat, save the meal and offer it at the next scheduled snack or meal. Missing an occasional meal will do no harm.

- **Watch for excess juice or milk intake.** Back to the previously made statement: juice is not a necessary part of the diet. This is the age group where parents often fall into the "juice trap." If you offer occasional juices, dilute them with water by at least half. Look for 100 percent fruit juices or buy fresh, refrigerated juices. Four to six ounces of juice per day is plenty. Dairy intake to fulfill calcium requirements in this age group is met if they consume 16 to 24 ounces of dairy products per day. Excess milk intake can lead to iron deficiency anemia because the toddlers are limiting so many other food choices and not getting adequate iron. Children who drink excess juice or milk can suppress their appetites with the fluids, and then not eat much at mealtime. If your child tends to guzzle 8 ounces of milk when he sits for the meal and then hardly eats, try offering only 3 or 4 ounces of milk at mealtime and then offer water. Soft drinks should not be a part of a toddler's diet.

- **Wean off the bottle.** This should be accomplished by 12 to 15 months of age. Research shows that bottle-weaning is later than expected among working mothers and that 42 percent were still bottle-fed after 2 years of age. This late bottle-feeding increases the risk of dental cavities and obesity later in life.[60] Toddlers often drink excess fluids with the bottle because it is easy and fast.

- **Allow your toddler the opportunity to exercise.** Toddlers need to be active, and in most cases, there is a natural instinct to run, play hide-and-seek, climb all over the furniture, and jump on the bed. However, today's lifestyles allow for a lot of sedentary activities that may limit toddlers' right to exercise. Television, videos, video games, and computers can limit their time for activity. Toddlers need to learn that it is fun to be active. We know that a lack of exercise and activity will lead to a higher risk of obesity. Set limits on television and computer time. (See p. 126 "Television-Watching Guidelines.") If you are the type of family that sits in the evening and watches two hours of television, try to schedule that time after your toddler is in bed. Going to the park or enrolling in a toddler gym program can create opportunities for exercise.

- **Don't use food to keep toddlers quiet or occupied.** This is a tough rule to follow, but if toddlers receive handouts at any moment of crisis, they start to see this as their reward. Avoid using food in the car to keep toddlers occupied. Of course, on a long car trip, appropriate planned snacks are fine, but using snacks for regular short trips around town can add a lot of extra calories to your toddler's diet. Avoid giving handouts when children are fighting with one another or during temper tantrums. Avoid giving snacks as "something to do" in response to boredom. It's better to plan for down time by bringing toys or books.

- **Junk food and fast food.** From the toddler stage forward, children will recognize fast food signs before they can read. They will learn from other children the names of foods that you have not heard of. I don't feel it is reasonable to never allow junk food or fast foods, but it is important to have some limits. An occasional outing to a fast food franchise is fine. However, you need to watch how often this is happening. The same goes for treats like candy, chips, and cookies. Use high-sugar and high-fat foods only as an occasional part of your children's diet, not as a regular routine. Research shows that repeated experience eating foods high in fat or sugar can predispose children to prefer these foods over foods like fruits and vegetables.[61]

- **Be a good role model.** Toddlers love to imitate. If they see their parents snacking on chips, eating fast foods frequently, and indulging in high-calorie desserts every night, they will follow suit. Look at your own eating habits. Having a child is a great reason to improve your own eating habits.

Chapter Eight
roundup
Toddlers: One to Three Years

- The more pressure put on toddlers to eat, the less they will probably eat.

- Relax about the amount of food your toddler eats! Make eating fun and low-key.

- Have family meals and offer regularly timed snacks and meals.

- Don't be a short-order cook for your toddler by going back in the kitchen to prepare other food choices.

- Don't bribe or reward with food.

- Don't use food as a distraction.

- Wean off the bottle by 12 to 15 months of age.

- Focus on healthy, fresh foods. Use fewer processed foods.

- It's fine to have occasional less healthy foods, but don't make them a way of life. Don't place a lot of emphasis on them as being special or forbidden.

- Follow your toddler's growth during regular checkups. If you have concerns about your toddler being overweight or underweight, discuss this with your pediatrician.

- Be an example! Change your own eating habits so that you can be a good role model.

nine
Chapter Nine
Preschoolers: Three to Five Years

What an enchanting age! The world around preschoolers is a giant discovery toy. Everything is a new adventure that they want to share with you. Communication skills are finally in place, and preschoolers have become a little more reasonable, pleasant, and fun to be with. They can now express themselves; much of their earlier frustration is gone.

Preschoolers understand the rewards of delayed gratification (although they may complain about it). They can communicate their needs and desires (although they don't always align with the parents' needs and desires). They are learning new skills and ideas at an incredible pace. They generally have a desire to please, and they understand feelings and may be vulnerable to having their own feelings hurt. One of the most popular lines a preschooler can injure with is "You're not invited to my birthday party." They are developing social skills and are not necessarily terrors at social outings. They are highly influenced by role models: parents, relatives, friends, television and movie characters, sports idols, and anybody else they take a general liking to. They still need limits and rules, but hopefully are testing less frequently.

When it comes to eating, they are learning new social skills and manners. "Please" and "thank-you" can become expected words. We can have them wash their hands before meals, come to the table, and even engage in some social conversation. They are able to handle their utensils and food without much help and without making a huge mess. (Yes, there will be the occasional spills and accidents, but at least they shouldn't be throwing their food by this stage.) They can actually help in the kitchen with some small tasks. At the end of this period, they can share in some responsibilities like helping to set and clear the table. They still come to the table with their likes and dislikes. Their dislikes may be as nit-picky as the way you cut their vegetables or that the vegetables are touching the rice.

As with toddlers, you are in charge of providing the food, and they are in charge of regulating how much they eat. According to research from the U.S. Department of Agriculture gathered from 1994 to 1996:

> Much of the decline in diet quality for children occurs between the age groups two to three and four to six. During this period, the percentage of children having a good diet falls from 35 to 16 percent, and the percentage having a diet that needs improvement rises from 60 to 75 percent.

This is an important age group for feeding! They are open to more social influences. How parents handle those influences may have a great impact on their eating choices years down the line. Many of the same tips for feeding and healthy foods from the toddler chapter apply to preschoolers, so review those if you haven't read them recently. In this chapter we will cover a few issues that are more unique to preschoolers.

Healthier Food Substitutes

Learn to read labels and weed out choices with too much sugar and fat and try to avoid the trans fats (see Chapter 3). The school-age child should be on the adult heart-healthy diet. You can make healthier food choices. Some are listed below. Many of the healthier suggestions and brands will be found at health food stores and will have fewer additives and colorings than their unhealthy counterparts. Ingredients are not listed here; do your own comparison-shopping to see the difference.

Instead of . . .	Try . . .
Cereals high in sugar	Oatios, Arrowhead Mills Nature Puffs, Health Valley Bran O's, Barbara's Fruity Punch Cereal
Hot dogs containing nitrates	Shelton's Turkey Franks (frozen section, no nitrates)
Packaged macaroni and cheese	Annie's Macaroni and Cheese
Tomato ketchup with sugar	Westbrae Natural Catsup
Peanut butter containing sugar or hydrogenated oils	Arrowhead Mills Organic Peanut Butter; also try almond butter, cashew butter
Jelly and jam	Cascadian Farm Organic Spreadable Fruit

Instead of . . .	Try . . .
Cheese type puffs	Little Bears Organic Lite Cheddar Puffs
Cookies	Westbrae Dino Snaps, Hain Animal Cookies
Hamburgers, hot dogs	Lean chicken, fish, vegetable or soy burgers
Chicken nuggets	Chicken fajita
Beef burrito with cheese	Bean burrito with rice, lettuce, tomato
Thick crust pepperoni pizza	Thin crust vegetarian pizza
Chips, tortilla chips	Air-popped popcorn, low-fat microwave popcorn, pretzels, baked tortilla chips, homemade pita chips
Crackers	Air-baked crackers, whole-grain crackers (Ak-Mak), rice cakes
Bologna	Low-fat turkey, chicken slices; better yet, use homemade chicken in sandwiches
Ranch dip	Bean dip, hummus, eggplant dip, yogurt
Meats	Tofu
French fries, instant potatoes	Baked potatoes, homemade oven fries, mashed potatoes with yogurt or buttermilk
Doughnuts, toaster pastries, croissants	Whole-grain bread, bagels, English muffins, pancakes or waffles with fruit
Cookies, cupcakes, brownies, cake	Graham crackers, fat-free fig bars, low-fat cookies
Ice cream	Low-fat frozen yogurt, fruit popsicles, sherbet
Milk shakes	Fruit and yogurt shakes

Great Eating Tips
for Preschoolers

(Review the feeding tips for toddlers, as many apply to the preschoolers.)

- **The one-bite rule.** Although preschoolers may be more willing than toddlers to try new food, this can still be a challenge. There is a technique called the "one-bite rule" that many families incorporate. I find that many preschoolers can follow this rule. The one-bite rule allows preschoolers to try the food, and if they do not like it, they do not need to finish it. My son, who loved the croutons in salads, was always encouraged to also take a bite of the lettuce. One night he asked for more salad, and at the age of four he turned into a great salad eater. Some children may adamantly refuse this rule, and then it is probably not worth the battle. Encourage, but never force. When your child has his fourth birthday, this could be one of the new rules for being four. Another trick to gain cooperation is to engage the help of your pediatrician. You could privately ask that at your child's next visit, the doctor discuss the "one-bite rule." I tell children that their taste buds change and food that did not taste good when they were three, may taste good when they are four. Sometimes hearing it from an authority can have an impact. They can keep a "New Food Diary" where they draw a picture of all the new foods they tried. They can label those they ended up liking. This could be sent to their doctor or any other important figure in their life.

- **The dinner choices.** Use varieties of fruits and vegetables at the dinner table. Many people do not think of offering fruits at dinner, but this can be an effective way to get vitamins and minerals into the child's diet. There are a lot of shared vitamins and minerals between the fruits and vegetables, so if your child is picky with the veggies, at least if he chooses some fruits, you have accomplished something. Try offering one or two choices of fruits and two choices of vegetables at the meal. If zucchini was refused once, still offer it a week or two later. They may change their mind.

- **Allow your children to help choose, prepare, and grow food.** Children who help pick out fruits and vegetables in the store and then help to prepare them may be more likely to eat them. Choose a new fruit, vegetable, grain, or legume to try. Depending on the age of the child, allow them to wash, break, or chop some foods. Involve them in menu planning and when appropriate, cooking. Another fun and educational activity for children is to grow their own vegetables. If you have a vegetable garden with small amounts of a large variety, some favorites may come to light. (See Appendix VII for resources on getting kids started with gardening.)

- **Allow your children to experiment with different dressings and dips.** Let them choose a dressing that suits their taste. These dressings can also become dips for favorite vegetables. Use yogurt dips and bean dips (homemade ones with white beans or garbanzo beans and a small amount of oil and garlic can be healthy and nutritious). Use a small amount of peanut butter or melted cheese as alternative dips. Add plain yogurt to fattier dips, like ranch, to "lighten" them. Try dips with yogurt and pureed fruits for a fruit dip.

- **Talk to your children about healthy eating.** At this age they can understand the concept of healthy eating. Discuss how healthy foods keep us healthy, and teach them about vitamins and minerals. Borrow books from the library about good foods, and the body and how it works. Ask them questions about the books. Role play (but not at the dinner table) different ways they handle being offered foods they don't like. Instead of "yuck," have them practice saying, "Sure, I will try a bite and see if I like it."

Books For Kids

Here a few favorite books about eating healthy:

The Berenstain Bears and Too Much Junk Food,
by Stan and Jan Berenstain (Turtleback, 1985)

D.W. the Picky Eater, by Marc Brown
(Little, Brown, 1995)

Green Eggs and Ham, by Dr. Seuss
(Random House, 1960)

Manners, by Aliki (Greenwillow, 1990)

Pyramid Pal, by Susan Norton and Susan Dawson
(Griffin Publishing, 2000)

The Race Against Junk Food, by Anthony Buono, Roy Nemerson, and Brian Silberman (HCOM Inc, 1994)

What Happens to Your Food? by Alastair Smith
(EDC Publications, 1997)

- **Watch the weight gain during this period.** Studies have shown that the odds of being obese as an adult were greater for children who were obese between the ages of 1 and 6. These odds were even higher if the child was obese at ages 10 to 14.[62] We do not want to have young children being paranoid about their weight or actively dieting (unless under a physician's care). However, some children who are identified as being overweight at this age can be helped with some simple early intervention. Limiting food and pressuring them to eat less is not appropriate in this age group. Try to make healthier choices. Doing things like cutting empty-calorie juices and sodas, going to non-fat or 1 percent milk, and limiting access to high-calorie snacks can be helpful. (See Chapter 12 for further suggestions on weight management.) Speak to your pediatrician if you have concerns about excess weight gain in this age period. Look at growth charts so you can see changing trends in children's weight gain. (See Appendix I, "Growth Charts.")

- **Encourage activity.** As mentioned in the previous chapter, sedentary activities like television, videos, video games, and computers need to be limited. In addition, children in this age group are highly influenced by television advertising (see following box). Activity is key to having a healthy preschooler. This promotes a natural way to burn energy and limits excessive weight gain. Make a point to walk with your preschoolers to places, go to the park, play outside, and encourage them to have fun with sports. Getting involved in sports can become the basis for preschoolers to establish a healthy lifestyle. They may start to enjoy learning new sports and getting involved in organized activities like soccer, T-ball, dance, gymnastics, basketball, and so forth. Have your child get involved because it's fun. Some kids aren't comfortable and ready for organized activities at this age. Don't force them to participate. Try to find physical activities that are compatible with the child.

Television-Watching Guidelines

- The American Academy of Pediatrics recommends a maximum of one to two hours a day of good-quality TV and video or computer games **combined.** On weekdays, I would recommend one hour a day combined or, better yet, none at all.

- Choose public television over commercial programming.

- Tape programs for children and fast-forward through commercials.

- Have a library of favorite videos or check them out from the video store.

- Some television channels do not run any advertising for foods or products.

- Avoid having a television set in the child's room.

- Watching television is a passive activity. The majority of programming does not promote physical, mental, social, or personal development. It is primarily a commercially driven medium that does not have the betterment of the child in mind.

- Television often creates unrealistic expectations in the mind of the child and creates an appetite for passive entertainment, junk food, and name brand "must-haves."

- Research shows that violent programs and computer games can lead to more aggressive behavior in children. Viewing repeated acts of violence desensitizes their perception of violence. Even during family programs, commercials may show violent previews for other programs and movies. With more concerns about real-life violence in children and teens, it gives us more reason to be mindful parents about the content and time spent watching television.

- **Remember: Excess television viewing equals lack of physical exercise, which leads to a higher risk for obesity.**

- **Talk about advertising.** Your preschooler who is watching television suddenly runs to you and says, "I want that! I want that!" He excitedly points to some sugary cereal or toy being advertised. Television advertising has a great influence on preschoolers. They see ads for unhealthy foods and for all the fast food restaurants in town. It has been estimated that 80 percent of advertisements in Saturday morning programming featured foods that were low in nutritional value.[63] Commercials for meat, dairy, bread, and juice make up only 4 percent of food ads. When was the last time we saw a commercial for spinach or carrots? Commercials for fruits and vegetables are almost nonexistent. It is important that we as parents recognize these influences, and first, avoid falling into the trap of buying all these kid-oriented foods, and second, discuss that these choices are less healthy ones.

  In 1994, Dr. Dale Kunkel from the University of California, Santa Barbara, found that children below the age of five could not discriminate between programs and advertisements. Children below seven to eight years of age do not recognize the persuasive intent of television advertising. Be discriminating both as a parent and a consumer, and explain to your child why you make certain choices. Be firm in not buying the latest unhealthy fad food just because it is requested.

- **Examine your food environment and buying habits.** This goes along with being a good role model. The food environment a parent provides influences the children's preferences and food acceptance. If there is a plate of cookies or a candy jar on the table, their cue to eat those foods is visually present. Keep tempting foods in the pantry to avoid the habit of snacking when not hungry. Remember, you are the parent, and you are in control of the environment.

- **Examine the daycare or preschool environment.** Find out what foods are being offered as snacks and meals and how often snacks are offered. Menus that change frequently offer the opportunity for children to experience new tastes. Also, ask about the policy on juices. Some daycares may allow juice at all times, but excess juice provides empty calories. If you are packing lunch for your preschooler, shop for healthier choices. (See p. 131 "Healthy Brown Bag Ideas.") In one study, preschoolers who didn't like certain foods showed an interest in choosing these foods after they observed other children selecting and eating them.[64] If you have an at-home caregiver, discuss your wishes about eating choices. If your caregiver is offering food that is in your home, it should be easy to control and monitor what is happening. If they take your child out for meals, make it clear how often you are comfortable with less healthy fast food choices. Providers who force children to "clean their plate" or use food as a reward or punishment are less likely to help children develop healthy eating habits.

- **Eating out: The Children's Menu.** When was the last time you looked at the children's menu and saw choices of vegetables or salads? The typical choices are hot dogs, chicken fingers, pizza, hamburgers, and french fries. Why not order a healthy appetizer off the adult menu or share an "adult" menu choice with your child or between kids? Before your child can read, you can be in control of the choices. Because eating out is a frequent occurrence with many families, the limited choices from a child's menu could be eaten three or four times a week for some children. Moderation is the key. Allow some outings where the choices may be off the children's menu, but if eating out is a frequent happening, select healthier choices from the adult menu.

- **Juice and sodas.** A small serving of juice may be offered as part of a snack or meal. Use 100 percent juice or citrus juices. Squeeze your own orange juice. Water should be the beverage of choice. Juice boxes are convenient for lunches and on-the-go drinks, but a water bottle works well, too. Four to six ounces of juice a day is plenty for preschoolers. Sodas should not be part of their diet.

- **Popeye eats spinach and that's what makes him strong.** Preschoolers are greatly influenced by role models. Kids who watch Popeye may try spinach. If only Tiger Woods could do cool commercials for healthy foods! If your child has a favorite role model, you could talk about how that role model must eat lots of broccoli for strong bones, or lots of carrots to see the ball well, or whatever else you want to encourage your child to eat. Preschoolers may eat this food choice because of what you said. It's worth a try.

- **Work on their table manners.** This is the age to work on several skills that should be achieved by the time children are four to five. They can say "please" and "thank you." They can learn to use a napkin and utensils properly and chew with the mouth closed. They can help set and clear the table. They should not whine or complain at the table. The child should be expected to sit throughout the meal and ask to be excused at the end. As with other aspects of parenting in this age group, limits must be set and clear expectations about behavior should be established. If you are having a hard time doing this in other aspects of your child's life, you will have difficulty at mealtime. Consult your pediatrician if you have concerns about your discipline efforts. A great book for kids, *Manners*, by Aliki, will teach them good etiquette.

Chapter Nine
roundup
Preschoolers: Three to Five Years

- Allow your child full control of how much to eat.
- Do not pressure, force, or insist on so many bites before dessert.
- Do not show concern about how much your child eats.
- Use regularly timed meals and snacks of healthy foods.
- Offer a variety of fresh foods.
- Try the "one-bite rule" for new foods.
- Allow your child to help choose or prepare food.
- Talk to your child about healthy eating and about advertisements.
- Encourage activity and exercise.
- Examine your own eating habits and food environment.
- Don't limit your child to the children's menu. Offer healthier choices from the adult menu.
- Develop expectations about behavior at mealtime.

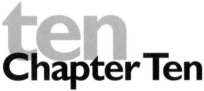

Chapter Ten
Elementary School Age Children

Once children go off to school, their world of influence grows and grows. What classmates—Billy, Jenny, Eric, and Robin—say, do, and bring in their lunches becomes very important to your child. Then there are the older children, the teacher, the librarian, the school nurse, the music teacher, the playground supervisor, the bus driver, the principal, and the cafeteria staff. Yes, your school child is faced with many choices and influences away from home.

Hopefully, if your child has developed skills of independence and learned to accept responsibility for behavior, your school age child has now turned into a positive and curious creature. In the early stages of this period, they are learning many new concepts in school and new social skills. They recognize that some children are better at some skills like art, sports, or reading. How they determine their self-worth when comparing themselves to other children will shape how they feel about themselves.

Over the last few years, if you have followed the principles of setting a good example and given your children good choices as they have been presented in the previous chapters, you may now see the benefits of your positive attitude about feeding. Your grade school children will become more independent and responsible about their eating. They will learn how to make their own breakfast and choose their own snacks. They will have their opinions about restaurants and the way food is prepared. They may even criticize your cooking! There are more situations where they are on their own and making their own decisions. You can pack a wonderful lunch and see most of it come home later that day. What happened? Did your child decide to eat a friend's lunch, buy lunch instead of eating what you had prepared, or maybe only took two bites and then went off to the playground?

Birthday parties and soccer or baseball games present more opportunities to eat less healthy foods. There is not much you can do to control these issues, and all of the above scenarios will probably happen.

Here are a few facts about school age children:

- Fifty percent of 5-year-old children consumed less than 2 servings of fruits and vegetables per day.[65]

- The prevalence of overweight among children between the ages of 6 and 17 has more than doubled in the past 30 years.

- Children who were overweight at age 7 were more likely to have multiple risk factors for heart disease as an adult. There was greater risk for having increased insulin levels, high blood pressure, and high cholesterol. Reduction in the *rate* of weight gain during childhood or adolescence had the potential to reduce the levels of young adult cardiovascular risk.[66]

Snacks

Create a snack plan for your children. List foods that are allowed anytime, sometimes, and occasionally for snacks as in the chart below. Post them on the refrigerator. Some suggestions for the different categories follow.

Anytime Snacks	Sometime Snacks	Occasional Snacks
Fruits	Cheese	Chips
Vegetables	Nuts	Candy
Low-fat yogurt	Dried fruit	Cakes
	Popcorn (use grated cheese, not salt and butter)	Cookies
	Low-fat crackers or pretzels	

Healthy Brown Bag Ideas

Below are some suggestions for packing a healthy lunch for school.

- Organic peanut butter sandwich wedges with jelly or honey. Add raisins, sliced bananas, strawberries, applesauce, grated carrots, or grated zucchini to the peanut butter.

- Bake a chicken in the beginning of the week, shred and slice it to use for lunches the rest of the week. This is a lot healthier than using processed lunch meats.

- Ask at your grocery store deli counter if they have meats in the case that do not have nitrates.

- Rolled-up tortillas filled with a thin layer of cream cheese and chicken or fish or filled with rice, beans, and cheese.

- Whole wheat pita breads with turkey, chicken, beans, grated vegetables, and rice.

- Use whole grain breads instead of white bread.

- Hard-boiled eggs or egg salad sandwiches. Add grated vegetables to the egg salad.

- Add chopped spinach, tomatoes, cucumbers, and a favorite dressing to pasta for a cold pasta salad. Tortellini filled with spinach and a touch of olive oil or flaxseed oil.

- Make a cold rice salad by chopping up vegetables, pineapples, apples, chicken, or fish and adding to rice.

- Use leftovers from dinner. Plan to make extra servings of healthy dinners to pack for lunches the next day.

- Pretzels, whole wheat crackers, bread sticks, or baked chips, are better than potato chips or corn chips.

- Offer graham crackers, fig bars, or oatmeal raisin cookies instead of chocolate chip cookies, cupcakes, or brownies.

- Yogurt. Avoid aspartame and sugary sprinkles.

Recipe Ideas

Healthy Brown Bag Squeezable Yogurts

Mix plain yogurt with puréed fruit. Add raisins, seeds, nuts (avoid these if concerned about choking hazards), or carob chips. Place in a snack-size plastic bag, freeze, pack for lunch, tear off a corner and eat. It is a healthy alternative to *Gogurts* and helps keep the lunch box cold.

Yogurt Dip For Fruits

1 tablespoon packed brown sugar or honey

1/2 teaspoon ground cinnamon

Dash of ground nutmeg

12 ounces vanilla yogurt

Mix all of the above and serve with cut-up fresh fruit.

Recipe Ideas

Frozen Popsicles

Any combination of fruits: berries, bananas, watermelon

12 ounces of seltzer water

1/2 cup orange juice

1/2 cup yogurt, optional

Blend and freeze in small paper cups with a popsicle stick inserted or in an ice cube tray or plastic Popsicle makers.

Oatmeal Raisin Cookies

1 cup whole wheat flour

3/4 cup wheat germ

1/2 cup rolled oats

3/4 tablespoon baking powder

2 teaspoon ground cinnamon

1 cup apple juice concentrate

1/4 cup vegetable oil

2 egg whites or 1 whole egg

3/4 cup raisins

Preheat oven at 375 F. Spray cookie sheet with vegetable cooking spray. Mix the first five ingredients in a large mixing bowl. Combine the juice concentrate, oil, egg, and raisins in a blender. Blend at medium speed until the raisins are chopped. Pour the mixture into the dry ingredients and stir together. Drop the batter by heaping teaspoons onto the prepared sheets, about 1 inch apart. Flatten with the back of a fork. Bake about 8 to 10 minutes. Cool.

- Any fresh fruits. Always try to pack at least one for lunch. Try whole or cut-up fruits.

- Pack carrots, celery, cucumber, green peppers, or soybeans (boiled edamame). Add a dip, peanut butter or light cream cheese.

- Pack a sticker, friendly picture, or note in your child's lunch to let them know you love them!

Great Eating Tips
for School Age Children

(Review the last chapter because many of those suggestions still apply to this older group of children.)

- **At home.** You still control many factors when your child is at home. What you buy and prefer to eat at home has a tremendous influence on the still-developing food choices of your school age child. Create a healthy food environment and your child will likely follow suit. Examine your cooking style and try to make necessary changes for healthy cooking. Use less butter and salt, limit meats—all family members will probably benefit from a healthy style of cooking.

  Remember the cardinal rule: you can't control how much your children eat or force them to eat and finish all their food. The one-bite rule mentioned in the previous chapter can be a way to encourage trying new foods, but respect the child's desire to cooperate with this rule. It should not be forced. They should not be bribed to take bites of food with sweet rewards. Trying foods should be a matter-of-fact occurrence, and their rejection or acceptance of the food should be met in a neutral fashion.

  Try to have meals as a family and allow for pleasant socializing. If meals turn into a time for nagging, criticizing or tension between you and your spouse, children don't eat as well. School age children have developed a lot of sophistication about parental tension and relationship problems. Unpleasant or difficult issues between the spouses, between adults and children, or between siblings should be dealt with away from mealtime. Family meetings scheduled once a week (away from mealtime) are opportunities for family members to air their concerns about issues and try to seek solutions. At the end of the meeting, have everyone say something positive about other family members.

- **Eating away from home.** As children go through these years, they will find themselves in many situations in which they will have to decide for themselves what and how much food to eat. Opportunities for buying their own food and snacks, and for eating at a friend's house and at parties, will create times for them to make their own decisions. Friends and peers will influence them along the way. Realize that these decisions must be allowed. A birthday party with a few hours of junk food isn't worth getting annoyed about. If they come home with a party bag full of candy, put most of it away and save it for an "occasional" snack.

- **The kitchen environment.** Keeping healthy snacks available is key to making eating healthy easy. It is often worth the extra trouble to wash fruits right after you buy them. Keep a special container at eye level in the refrigerator filled with a variety of cut-up vegetable choices. A container with several compartments that has a sealed lid is easy. Make a fruit salad every couple days and the fruit will usually disappear faster. Take fruit that is "near the end" and use it in smoothies or make fruit popsicles. Have a moratorium on certain foods. Why have potato chips or tortillas in the house constantly? We probably eat enough of that at parties and restaurants. Stop buying a few favorite junk foods for a while. You may be surprised that they are not missed that much. Keep the high-fat and high-sugar snacks out of sight and less accessible to little hands.

- **Spending money.** If you find your child is spending much of his or her allowance on unhealthy food, then maybe it's time to discuss how you manage the family budget. You can explain that a certain percentage goes to food, a percentage goes to savings, a percentage goes to charity, etc. Children can start to learn the principles of money management.

- **School lunch.** Many schools have choices offered by popular fast food restaurants. Even if some of these offer more healthful choices, what type of message is this sending our children? Carefully examine your child's school lunch program, and if you are not satisfied, voice any complaints. Change won't occur if parents are not involved. Consult the *Healthy School Lunch Action Guide* by Susan Campell and Todd Wirant if you are interested in changing your local school's lunch program. (See Appendix VII.) If packing a lunch has become a way of life from the beginning of your child's school attendance, it may be easier to continue the pattern. Of course, a packed lunch is only as healthy as you make it.

Allow your children to be involved with the shopping and the packing of lunches. If your children want to buy lunch at school, negotiate a reasonable number of times per week this is allowed, especially if your school lunch program is offering less-than-healthy foods.

- **After-school snacks.** Set up guidelines for after-school snacks. (See p. 131, "Anytime, Sometimes, and Occasional

Snacks.") If it is too close to dinner, allow only anytime snacks. When I prepare dinner I set out a bowl of carrot sticks and my son knows that these are "anytime snacks" that he can nibble on before dinner.

- **Cooking and shopping.** Find a local cooking class for children. Teach them how to plan meals and have them write up a menu for the week. Allow them to get involved with shopping. Make a list and stick with it at the store. This will teach them not to be tempted by the latest fad foods and impulsive buying at the market. Teach them how to read nutrition labels. Use the grocery store as an educational tool. Set up a time of the week, like Sunday afternoons to cook some healthy snacks or cookies that will be available during the week for the family. It can be a time to reconnect with your kids and start a new tradition.

- **Talk about how food choices and the environment affect health.** The school age child is now sophisticated enough to learn about the body and how food choices may affect health. On a simple level, you can explain how protein gives you muscles, calcium gives you strong bones, and fruits and vegetables give you vitamins that fight illness. As they get older, you can discuss calcium and osteoporosis, how the American Cancer Society recommends five fruits and vegetables a day to reduce the risk of developing cancer, how fatty foods clog blood vessels and lead to heart attacks. Teach your children about the environment and recycling and how a healthy environment will help to ensure a healthy future. Discuss organic foods.

- **Those loving relatives.** Sometimes there are family members other than the mother and father involved in raising and feeding the children. Aunts, uncles, and grandparents may have active roles in feeding your children. Relatives may also be frequent visitors in your home and offer advice and sometimes criticism about the way you should or should not feed your children. If your children are receiving special treats on occasion from loving relatives, but they maintain a general good diet, relax. If relatives are highly involved in feeding of your children and you see many unhealthy choices being offered, it may be time to seek words of wisdom from another source. Taking the relative to the child's annual physical exam and letting your pediatrician know your concerns may be helpful. This is important if there is a weight problem developing. Advice from the doctor may sound less like criticism to a caring relative. There are plenty of short articles found in many parenting magazines that address the value of healthy eating. Share that information with them. Share parts of this book and other books on healthy eating habits with them. (See Appendix VII, "Suggested Reading and Web Sites.") If you act like you are trying to acquire their help in keeping your kids healthy and not find fault with them, they are more likely to listen.

- **Concerns about weight.** As children progress through these years, there may be concerns about weight—from the child or the parents. If children are slightly chubby and worried about their weight, try to make them feel comfortable about their body image. Even if they are markedly overweight, let them know they are still special! Having family members accuse a child of being fat is destructive to their self-esteem. An exam with a doctor to look at growth charts and the trend for weight gain is a good way to find out how your child is really doing. (See p. 147, "Defining Overweight and Obese.") Studies show that children who are overweight by age nine will likely remain overweight through the next several years. Overweight children were also found to have a higher blood pressure and cholesterol than their lighter peers.[68] (See Chapter 12 for suggestions on weight management.)

Chapter Ten
roundup
Elementary School Age Children

- Continue to follow the cardinal rule about food: no forcing, coaxing, or nagging.

- Offer healthy choices, and allow children to decide how much and what to eat.

- Create a snack plan of "anytime," "sometimes," and "occasional" foods.

- Read labels and look for healthier choices.

- Buy foods that have lower fat, lower sugar, and fewer additives and preservatives.

- Control the food environment at home.

- Relax about food opportunities away from home.

- Examine your child's school lunch program, and decide with your child what is reasonable for packed lunches and the frequency of buying lunch.

- Shop for groceries with your children and teach them how to read labels. Enroll your children in healthy cooking classes, and encourage their involvement in menu planning and cooking.

- Identify any serious weight problems with the help of your pediatrician and address problems of excess weight gain.

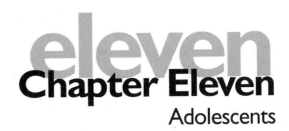

Chapter Eleven

Adolescents

Teenagers have been described as "toddlers with hormones and wheels."

Toddlers have been described as "going through their first adolescence."

Toddlers and adolescents have some common traits. They are both learning to be individuals and appear rebellious, negative, and defiant along the way. Both are transition stages: one is from babyhood to childhood and the other from childhood to adulthood.

The "Terrible Two's" and adolescence are often the dreaded stages of development. However, if they are handled with loving authority and respect for who the child is and why the child has to go through these stages, you don't have to dread them at all. In fact, you can really enjoy them.

The defiance parents face when they deal with adolescents is necessary for teenagers to create their own identity. Realize that a large part of what is shaping your teenager's actions today is based on what has occurred throughout his or her childhood. He or she has been shaped by your ideas, influences, and discipline, whether your teen wants to admit it or not. Now, this young adult will try to defy your ideas, influences, and discipline. But for the most part, your teen will eventually accept what you have been teaching all along.

The challenge to parents of adolescents is letting go and allowing freedom. It is also about respecting them and allowing them their opinions. Realize you have to pick your battles. Does this sound like a familiar statement from the toddler chapter?

Establish boundaries and limits, as you have in all other age groups, and allow their freedoms to be earned as they demonstrate they can handle them. It is time to play more of a support role than a controlling role. Being too authoritarian (the "I must know everything" approach) or too permissive (the "anything goes" approach) can cause troubled adolescents. If raising an adolescent sounds like you are on a teeter-totter, it is—one day you're the good guy, the next day you're the bad guy; one day your idea is brilliant, the next day it was a terrible idea.

As far as food issues, adolescents will have to be left to their own devices when away from the home environment. You can only hope that the lessons you have instilled from a young age will shine through, but adolescents will test the limits of eating. They may boast to their friends about how many candy bars or pancakes they ate at one sitting. The power of unsupervised eating is a limit that most adolescents try to test. Even though you may hear of these unwitnessed events, take heart! A recent study showed that teens were more influenced by what their family ate than what their friends ate. Fat intakes were more in line with the family's intakes than their peer group's fat intakes.[69] So you should keep up the modeling of healthy eating habits at home, and understand that teens need their freedom. They will take nutritional risks. Probably, if you reflect on your own teenage eating habits, you may recall a few outrageous food binges or habits. Maybe if you share some of those with your teen, you both can have a good laugh.

Here are some trends seen in teenagers.

- Research by the U.S. Department of Agriculture from 1994 to 1996 showed that 12 percent or less of adolescents ages 15 to 18 met the dietary recommendation for fruits. They also found a noticeable decline in diet quality between the 7 to 10 and 11 to 14 age groups, with the percentage of children having a good diet falling from 14 to 7 percent.

- In 1994, nearly three-fourths of teenage boys drank an average of 34 ounces (almost three 12-ounce cans) of soda per day. Two-thirds of teenage girls drank 23 ounces of soda per day. A 12-ounce can of regular soda contains nearly a quarter cup of sugar.

- Adolescent girls were unlikely to receive the minimum requirements of the Food Guide Pyramid. Adolescent boys were more likely to meet the requirements for grains, vegetables, and meats, though they tended to consume more fat than recommended. Adolescents who did not meet the Food Guide Pyramid are likely to be deficient in vitamin B-6, folic acid, calcium, iron, zinc, and fiber.

- A moderately active adolescent boy needs about 2,700 calories per day and a moderately active adolescent girl needs about 2,300 calories per day. Variation in activity and build will change these caloric intake numbers. A boy doing intense athletic activity may need up to 5,000 calories a day, and a sedentary girl may need only 2,000 calories a day.

Effective Communication with Adolescents

Although food issues are only one small part of the parenting package with adolescents, all issues with your teens must be handled with effective communication skills. The following are some quick tips.

- Pick your battles.
- Be specific.
- Be brief.
- Listen actively with your eyes and ears.
- Avoid giving too many orders and too much advice.
- Avoid threats, sermons, criticism, and ridicule.
- Create times without distractions where you are available to talk.

Vegetarian Diets

Vegetarians who understand nutrition and the combining of foods are healthier than their Western meat-eating counterparts. However, some adolescents embark on a vegetarian diet without understanding what they need to do to avoid nutritional deficiencies. The reason for adopting a vegetarian diet is usually because of sensitivity to the issue of eating animals. Most of the time, females are the ones who adopt a vegetarian diet.

Depending on how strict a vegetarian diet is being followed, nutritional deficiencies can occur. Strict vegetarians who avoid all meat and fish, dairy products, and eggs are at risk for vitamin B-12 deficiency, which can lead to anemia. Vitamin D deficiency may also be a problem if there is little sunlight exposure. Calcium is not as well absorbed from plant sources as from dairy products. Zinc deficiency may occur because the best sources of zinc are from yogurt, liver, and beef.

If your family is a meat-eating family and your teenager has decided to become vegetarian, it is best to educate your teenager to ensure adequate intake of needed nutrients. A nutritional supplement of vitamins and minerals with calcium is necessary. Trying to discourage a teenager who is set on vegetarianism will most likely cause a more rebellious attitude about eating. See the reference section in Appendix VII for books on vegetarian diets.

Nutritional Deficiencies

Adolescents are one of the most nutritionally deficient population groups. This is especially true of adolescent girls. This occurs at a time when they are growing rapidly and need good nutrition. A high quality nutritional supplement is important. The following section will address iron, calcium, and fiber needs in teens.

Iron

The function of iron in the body is to produce hemoglobin for the red blood cells. Iron deficiency is usually caused from insufficient intake, but other factors also deplete iron stores. These depleting factors include excess menstrual bleeding, chronic illnesses, excess coffee or tea consumption, and strenuous exercise. Teenagers, especially athletic teenagers, need extra iron. The RDA for iron for adolescent girls is 15 milligrams a day and 12 milligrams a day for boys, but it is higher for athletic teenagers. Iron absorption from foods in our diet is somewhere between 10 and 20 percent, depending on the food source. Taking foods rich in vitamin C at the same time as iron-rich foods can increase iron absorption by as much as 30 percent. Foods like tea, coffee, bran, and milk taken with iron foods can decrease iron absorption by as much as 50 percent.

Signs of iron deficiency include fatigue, dizziness, pallor, nervousness, and finally, anemia. If your teenager avoids meat, fish, poultry, and dark green leafy vegetables, he or she may be at risk for iron deficiency. A blood test will detect iron deficiency. Early on, a teenager can be iron deficient without showing anemia in a blood test. Looking at the size of the red blood cells and checking iron levels are a better way to detect early iron deficiency. If you suspect iron deficiency, discuss this with your teenager's doctor.

Calcium

A study from 1998 showed that only 19 percent of adolescents were aware of the RDA for calcium, and their average calcium intake was about 50 percent of the RDA.[70] Only 12 percent of girls between the ages of 15 and 18 met the dietary recommendation for dairy intake, according to statistics released from the U.S. Department of Agriculture. In 1997, the National Academy of Sciences recommended increasing the calcium requirements for teenagers to 1,300 milligrams per day. To receive this, a teenager needs to eat four daily servings of dairy (milk, cheese, ice cream, yogurt, or cottage cheese) plus a good serving of green vegetables. In addition, tofu, calcium-fortified soy milk, calcium-fortified rice milk, calcium-fortified orange juice, dark green leafy vegetables (like kale and collards), broccoli, soybeans, canned salmon with bones, and almonds are sources of calcium. The high phosphorus content of soft drinks decreases calcium absorption. Have your teens track their calcium intake for a few days to get an idea of their daily calcium intake. Many teenagers will discover that they need to take a calcium supplement to fulfill their requirements.

Fiber

Many teenagers have low fiber intake. This is primarily due to their decreased fruit and vegetable consumption. They should be receiving the recommended amount set for adults of 25 to 35 grams per day. Fiber goals will be met if they eat five servings of fruits (preferably whole, fresh fruit) and vegetables, two slices of whole wheat bread, a breakfast cereal with three or more grams of fiber, and one to two other servings of high fiber foods. (See Appendix II, "High Fiber Foods.")

The health benefits of fiber include reduces cholesterol, curbs overeating, keeps the intestines healthy, helps to avoid constipation, and reduces cancer risk.

Great Eating Tips
for Adolescents

- **Use meals as a time to be social.** Teens start to have other obligations and may not always make it to the family meal. Use family mealtime as a way to be social and catch up on news. Try not to use meals as a venue for stressful conversations or to settle problems. This is best done at a family meeting away from the dinner table. If your teens are not going to be home for dinner, it is reasonable for them to let you know where they will be eating.

- **Try to offer suitable, healthy, quick foods for snacks and breakfast.** Teens are often in a hurry and need quick and easy foods to grab for breakfast and snacks. Agree on some easy food choices to have available, and encourage them not to skip meals. Research has shown that kids who skip meals and are hungry had poorer performances on standardized testing.[71]

- **Allow teens to cook and menu plan.** With more working couples, placing a home-cooked meal on the table can be a challenge. Today, more couples share in the responsibility of cooking. Teens can also share in some of the responsibility of cooking and meal planning. If you've been asking them to share responsibility all along, this should not be a difficult request. Asking them to plan one meal a week either alone or with one parent is a way to keep them involved.

- **Maintain family eating rituals.** Traditions and rituals are an important part of growing up. In many families, holidays offer classic rituals revolving around meals. But family rituals can go beyond the holidays. Family picnics, Sunday breakfasts, or a traditional family meal on a certain night of the week can all be ways to reconnect. Teens have a tendency to want to spend less time with their families and more time with friends. They should be allowed to develop their friendships, but if there are important family events, make it clear that your teens are expected to participate.

- **Allow for nutritional errors.** Active teenagers can eat a lot of calories, especially boys. They have a larger margin for error in regard to consuming empty calories. Because of their increased calorie need, they can eat a larger percentage of nutritionally worthless food and still get most of their basic nutrients if some of the food they eat is nutritious. This does not mean a free license to eat junk food, but parents need to have a relaxed attitude about their teen eating occasional fast foods with friends or pounding down a candy bar with lunch.

- **Watch the caffeine intake.** A soda at lunch, a cafe latte after school, and then more coffee for study time in the evening can add up. A can of cola contains almost as much caffeine as a cup of coffee. With the popularity of coffee houses, teenagers are developing a taste for trendy coffee drinks. Many of these drinks are loaded with extra calories and fat. Watch for sources of caffeine that are not so obvious like *Sunkist Orange*, *Mountain Dew*, tea, chocolate, cocoa, and some over-the-counter pain relievers. Too much caffeine can cause jitteriness, a racing heart, heartburn, anxiety, and insomnia. If teenagers are used to a daily dose of caffeine, they can experience symptoms of withdrawal (headaches, stomach cramps, irritability, and depression) when they miss a day or two of it.

- **Let teens hear nutritional information from professionals.** Teens are often willing to hear and accept information from people other than their parents. Encourage them to take classes on nutrition and health or cooking classes. (Hopefully, they are getting some of this in school.) Buy them books about nutrition and health. Your teen's physician or a dietician can be helpful if you have serious concerns about nutrition.

- **Continue to encourage physical activity.** Strength training can be added to the teenage program of exercise; this is especially good for their bones and their metabolism. Many local gyms have teen exercise programs available. Some teenage girls, especially if they have a weight problem, are self-conscious and uncomfortable in a group setting. Renting or purchasing exercise videos can be an alternative. Exercising with a parent, friend, or sibling may help to motivate the adolescent. The key is scheduling exercise ahead of time and writing in on the calendar. Any type of organized sport or activity will be beneficial. In the summers, look for camp programs that encourage more active events.

Chapter Eleven
roundup
Adolescents

- Don't sweat the nutritional blunders that are likely to occur along the way.
- Encourage family meals when possible.
- Allow teens to menu plan and cook.
- Watch caffeine intake.
- Talk to a health professional about specific concerns such as obesity, eating disorders, and vegetarian diets.
- Encourage physical activities with team sports, individual activity at a gym or at home, or family-oriented physical activities.
- Learn to recognize possible deficiencies in iron, calcium, and a fiber. Educate your adolescent on these deficiencies and work together to find ways to fill in the gaps.

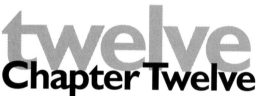

Chapter Twelve
Eating Problems:
Weight Management and Eating Disorders

Childhood obesity has reached epidemic proportions and is becoming a worldwide issue that will have serious healthcare implications as these children age. Because of struggles surrounding food, eating disorders are also becoming more common. These two seemingly opposite issues about weight are based on similar issues surrounding eating, pleasure, reward, and guilt.

Is Your Child Overweight?

Although this seems like it would have a simple answer, there are many different opinions on how to define "overweight" or "obese." The medical definitions are explained in the box below. Many parents do not recognize the weight issues with their child. They may perceive their child as being normal weight, when reality on the growth curve shows a problem. This is why regular check-ups with your child's doctor and identifying changes in weight gain can be very important. The odds of success are much higher if a child with a weight issue is managed early.

Is it in the Genes?

Although there does appear to be some genetic predisposition to obesity, lifestyle also has a tremendous impact on weight, too. Scientists have found genes may play a role in obesity. Studies have shown that if one parent is obese, there is a 40 percent chance and if both parents are obese, there is an 80 percent chance of the child being overweight. Adopted children tend to follow weight patterns similar to their biological parents and not their adoptive parents.

Research showing how environment influences weight becomes evident when different ethnic groups are examined. The Japanese are typically not prone to obesity, but Japanese-Americans are 15 to 20 pounds heavier than people in Japan. This discrepancy is explained by the different dietary practices in the two countries. Even societies that have traditionally not had many problems with obesity, like Japan, are seeing a rise in this pattern. From 1974 to 1995, the rate of childhood obesity among Japanese children has doubled from 5 to 10 percent.[72]

One important concept to recognize is that once a person becomes overweight, their fat cells secrete hormones that influence the metabolic rate. This cycle tends to increase the number of fat cells. It becomes harder to lose weight. This is why most people find it difficult to lose weight once they are overweight.

This should be a real incentive to address any overweight issues early, rather than later. It is easier and more effective to take this approach.

Defining Overweight and Obese

Clinically being "overweight" or "obese" in medical terms has been defined in adults, but less clearly defined in children. For adults, body mass index (BMI) is one way to determine whether or not you are overweight and by how much. BMI is calculated by multiplying weight in pounds by 703 and then dividing that number by height in inches squared.

$$BMI = weight\ (pounds) \times 703 \div height\ (inches)^2$$
$$OR$$
$$BMI = weight\ (kilograms) \div height\ (meters)^2$$

Body mass index may be overestimated in people who are muscular or athletic. According to definitions established by the National Heart, Lung, and Blood Institute, **"overweight"** is a BMI value between 25 and 29.9 and **"obesity"** is a BMI value greater than or equal to 30 for adults.

For children between 2 and 20 years of age, new BMI charts are now available that allow health professionals to identify children who are **"underweight,"** **"at risk"** for being overweight, and those children who are likely **"overweight."** The BMI value that is "appropriate" varies with the age; therefore percentiles are used to guide us.

Underweight	BMI for age <5th percentile
At risk of overweight	BMI for age ≥85th percentile
Overweight	BMI for age ≥95th percentile

Charts are available on the Internet on the Center for Disease Control website at www.cdc.gov/growthcharts/ and can also be found in Appendix I.

The BMI charts for children do have their limitations and should be used only as a guideline. Factors such as high levels of physical activity, early maturation, genetics, muscle mass, and bone structure can influence the BMI and may falsely identify a child as "at risk" for being overweight or being "overweight." Please consult your child's health professional for accurate interpretation of these growth curves and how it applies to your child. A high or low BMI is not always cause for concern.

Guidelines for Controlling Weight Problems in Children

The following are some suggestions for managing weight issues for kids.

- Check with your pediatrician about your child's height and weight first to determine if there is a significant problem. Sometimes, what may seem like a problem to the parent or the child is not a problem when looked at in perspective with past weight and height.

- Prevention is the key. Following growth throughout childhood can identify children at risk. If children are overweight before adolescence, the goal is to try to slow down weight gain. This way, as children gain in height, they will thin out.

- Have the whole family model healthy eating patterns. If the child is discouraged from certain food choices, but other family members are allowed those choices, the child will feel singled out as having a problem. Make healthy eating a family choice. If your child is always looking for "seconds," make a rule that no one gets "seconds" until everyone is done with "firsts." This may allow them more time to feel full.

- Choose low glycemic foods. Read the following section to learn more about this important concept for weight control.

- Don't calorie-restrict children. Don't take the message of dieting or low-fat or non-fat eating to the extreme. Don't obsess with your child over every fat gram and sugar calorie. The goal is to make better choices, but still fulfill a normal eating pattern.

- Avoid power struggles surrounding food. Forcing kids to eat certain foods or "clean your plate" will lead to problems and make eating an unpleasant event.

- Decrease fat intake, but don't let that fool you. With many lower fat choices of foods available, this is getting easier. However, even low-fat foods in excess quantities can lead to weight gain, and some low-fat foods are high in sugar. Avoid the fats labeled as "partially hydrogenated" or "hydrogenated."

- Don't forbid junk food, just use it less often. Do not buy the junk food like chips, soda, juice, cookies, candy, cake and ice cream to have in the house. Most families find themselves eating out enough that the kids will get these foods outside the home at restaurants, parties, or special occasions.

- Read the labels, especially for foods like cereals and snack foods.

- Limit fast foods to less than once every two weeks and find healthier fast food choices.

- Trim the fat off meats and avoid eating the chicken skin.

- Use low-fat cooking techniques at home.

- Eat five servings of fruits and vegetables a day and increase fiber intake.

- Cook only enough for a serving size for each family member.

- Use more grains, soy (like tofu), and beans instead of meats.

- Make water the beverage of choice over juice and soda.

- Use 1 percent or non-fat milk. It is best to try to make the switch to non-fat milk. Try mixing 1 percent with non-fat to start and then gradually wean out the 1 percent.

- Try a snack plan and set up the occasional foods to happen only 2 or 3 times a week. (See p. 131, "Snacks.")

- Encourage and find physical activities that the child enjoys.

- Limit television, computer, and video game time. It is best to eliminate or allow a maximum of $1/2$ to 1 hour of TV, video, or computer time a night for school nights. The exception may occur if the computer is needed for homework.

- Don't allow snacking in the car, in front of the television, or while doing homework.

- When eating out, share meals and try to avoid the unhealthier "kid meals." Ask for pizza with half the cheese or ask if low-fat cheese is available. Skip the cheese on burgers and eat only one half of the bread bun. Don't "supersize." Skip the mayonnaise on sandwiches.

- Make changes gradually. Change 1 or 2 poor eating habits into good habits at a time. If you try to make a lot of drastic changes, you will likely drive everyone in the family crazy and they will find their "junk food habit" somewhere else.

- Seek professional help with your pediatrician or nutritionist if you are having difficulty. (See Appendix VII.)

- Love and appreciate your children regardless of their size. Do not make negative comments about their weight. Avoid nagging, criticizing, or pressuring your children about food. Praise their efforts for trying to make positive changes in their eating habits.

Glycemic Index (GI)

High glycemic index (GI) foods release sugar into the bloodstream quickly, causing a rapid rise in blood sugar. *Low glycemic foods* release sugar into the bloodstream slowly and do not cause a rapid rise in blood sugar. High GI foods tend to lead to weight gain and are low in fiber. These foods are easy to overeat and encourage a rapid return of hunger. Low GI foods are less likely to store as fat and maintain more stable energy levels. Low GI foods also reduce the hunger urges by delaying the rate of absorption.

Interesting research is appearing on low glycemic diets as a way to manage pediatric obesity. A study from the *Archives of Pediatric & Adolescent Medicine* found that children on a low GI diet did better than children on a low-fat diet. Those on the low GI diet had better weight loss results and what was most striking was that this group did not need a reduction in serving sizes. They were able to eat until fullness and still lose weight.

Here are some guidelines for finding foods with a low or moderate GI:

- Most fruits and vegetables have a low GI. Bananas, beets, carrots, corn, and potatoes have a higher GI and should be chosen less often.

- Choose beans, legumes, soybeans.

- Choose lean meats, poultry, and seafood.

- Look for whole grain breads, other whole grains, and pastas with more protein content. (See p. 109, "The Goods on Grains.")

Glycemic Carbohydrates

High Glycemic Carbohydrates	Low Glycemic Carbohydrates
bananas	apples
cooked potatoes, all types	apricots
corn	barley
corn chips	brown rice
corn flakes	bulgur
crackers	fructose, lactose
french fries	grapes
honey, glucose	high fiber, whole grain cereals
jams	kiwi
low fiber, sugary cereals	legumes, especially lentils, chick peas, split peas, kidney beans, white beans, soy beans
millet	milk, skim milk, yogurt
orange juice	oranges
Puffed Rice and Puffed Wheat	peanuts
raisins	protein-enriched pastas
soft drinks	sourdough bread
white bread	strawberries
white rice, especially the instant type	whole-grain rye bread

Getting Active

Kids need to be active in order to help them manage their weight. Studies have shown that just turning off the TV in the house can lead to weight loss. Getting exercise does not mean that your child has to join every organized sports team. Organized sports can be a great way to keep kids active, but watch and see how active they are at practices and games. With some sports, actual "active" time may be limited to 5 or 10 minutes, with kids standing around, watching or listening to instructions instead of being active. We want to ensure that kids get "sweaty" activity just about every day.

Ways to get exercise for kids would include walking (how about going with mom and dad, so they can get their exercise in, too!), running, skateboarding (make sure they have their pads and helmet!), swimming, biking, and in-line skating. Schedule time for exercise with the family and write it down on the calendar. Chores can also be a way to burn some calories, like cleaning windows, shoveling snow, washing the car, gardening, vacuuming, and weeding. Other active ideas include hopscotch, Frisbee, inventing a dance, tag, badminton, balloon volleyball, jump roping, sprinting through the sprinkler, tumbling practice, and making angels in the snow.

Please see **www.kidseatgreat.com** for information on Dr. Wood's *Kids Weigh to Go* program.

Eating Disorders

Eating disorders affect over five million Americans, but this number is probably conservative. Many people hide their eating disorders. Anorexia nervosa with its drastic weight loss, and bulimia, which involves binging and purging, are the two well-recognized eating disorders. One study estimates that up to 20 percent of adults and teens have bulimia at some point in their lives. Most commonly, eating disorders involve females between the ages of 14 and 25, but younger girls, as well as males, are also being identified today. Eating disorders are characterized by a distortion about eating and an underlying emotional problem. People with eating disorders can be underweight, normal weight, or even overweight. They are obsessed with food and weight control issues.

Signs of an eating disorder can include a child or teenager who:

- skips meals, is "too busy" to eat, or insists on preparing her own low-fat meal
- is overly concerned about weight, and complains that she is too fat even if she is thin
- disappears into the bathroom after meals (a sign of laxative abuse or induced vomiting)
- has lost a lot of weight in a short time
- cooks high-fat foods for others, but refuses to eat any herself
- analyzes nutrition labels, calories, and fat grams
- exercises excessively, and often counts calories burned for every physical activity
- has physical signs like a disruption or absence of menstrual periods, dry skin, downy hair on the face and arms, constipation, rashes, and itching
- has erosion of tooth enamel due to self-induced vomiting
- has behavior changes like angry outbursts, withdrawn behavior, isolation from friends, depression, poor sleep patterns
- wears loose clothing to hide weight loss.

If your child or teenager shows a combination of these warning signs, seek professional help. These children need a team approach with nutrition counseling,

Chapter Twelve
roundup
Weight Management and Eating Disorders

psychotherapy, and appropriate medical care. See Appendix VII to find resources for eating disorders.

- Identify trends of increasing weight gain early and make dietary changes.

- Learn about high glycemic and low glycemic foods.

- Seek professional help if there are difficult eating issues, or your child is significantly overweight, or you suspect an eating disorder.

SECTION C

The War Against Diseases—Now & Long Into Adulthood

thirteen
Chapter Thirteen
Allergies, Asthma, and Eczema

Asthma is the fifth most common chronic illness in all ages and the most prevalent chronic condition among children. Between 1980 and 1994, there has been a 75 percent overall increase of asthma in the United States. In preschool children, there has been a 160 percent increase in the same time period. Children and adults over 65 are the two age groups with the most asthmatics.

Allergic rhinitis, commonly known as hay fever, affects 23.7 million Americans. Often, children with allergies and asthma have a family history of hay fever, asthma, or eczema. *Eczema* or *atopic dermatitis* affects about 10 percent of all infants and children.

These three processes are allergic or *atopic* and tend to run in families. They are allergic responses to pollens or other environmental stimuli (like dust, mold, smoke, air pollution, animal dander, and stress). Experts attribute this higher incidence to the rising levels of environmental pollution.

Reactive Airways Disease (RAD) or Asthma Symptoms

- Wheezing: The wheezing noted in asthmatics is a result of hypersensitivity of the airways to stimuli that causes a spasm or narrowing of the small airways of the lungs; when these airways narrow, wheezing is heard. It sounds like high-pitched whistling when audible, but it can sometimes only be heard with a stethoscope.

- Coughing: Some children cough as a symptom of their asthma and do not wheeze. These coughing episodes can be triggered by environmental exposure to elements like smoke. It can also be aggravated with exercise.

- Tightness in the chest or difficulty breathing.

Allergic Rhinitis (Hay Fever) Symptoms

- Itchy, watery eyes and nose

- Sneezing

- Thin, watery nasal discharge that may occur on and off

- Constant sniffling

- Clicking noises made with tongue against the roof of the mouth

- Dark circles under the eyes which are known as "allergic shiners"

- Horizontal crease across the middle of the nose from constant rubbing, known as an "allergic crease."

Eczema or Atopic Dermatitis (AD) Symptoms

- Usually begins in the first year of life and is often outgrown by grade school or adolescence

- Itchy, dry scaly, red rash

- Often involves the face, inner surface of elbows and knees folds.

Micronutrients and Allergies

What have researchers discovered about the link between allergic processes and nutrition? The following is a summary of some of this research. Most of these studies have been conducted in adults.

- Vitamin C is a major antioxidant substance in the airway surface liquid of the lung where it could be important in protecting against environmental oxidants. A study from the *American Journal of Clinical Nutrition* showed that a diet low in vitamin C was a risk factor for asthma.[73]

- Patients with asthma who reported a high dietary magnesium intake had better lung function and a reduction in the relative risk of wheezing.[74] Animal studies have shown that magnesium deficiency increases the amount of histamine released into the blood. Histamine is a natural chemical in our bodies that, when released, causes many of the symptoms of allergies.

- Low selenium levels were observed in patients with asthma when compared to a group of patients without asthma.[75]

- In a group of 20 patients with exercise-induced asthma, two grams of vitamin C was administered and lung function was tested. In nine patients, a protective effect on their exercise-induced asthma was documented after vitamin C was given.[76]

- A dietary questionnaire used to determine intakes of different nutrients in patients with asthma and allergic rhinitis, and then in control patients without disease, showed that those with the lowest intakes of vitamin C and manganese were associated with more than five-fold increased risk of asthma. Also those with low intakes of zinc had increased risk of symptoms of seasonal allergies, and those with low magnesium intakes had increased risk of asthma.[77]

- Children who ate fresh oily fish had a significantly reduced risk of asthma. No other food groups or nutrients were significantly associated with either an increased or reduced risk of asthma. This study concluded that consumption of oily fish might protect against childhood asthma.[78]

- A study of 17 adult asthmatics found that when their diets were supplemented with daily dosages of 400 IU of vitamin E and 500 milligrams of vitamin C there was an 18 percent increase in the peak flow capacity (a measure of lung function) over those on regular diets.[79]

- Proanthocyanidins (found in grape seed extract) have been found to have an antihistaminic effect.[80]

- Maternal diet rich in saturated fats during breastfeeding was found to sensitize infants to more atopic disease.[81]

- Researchers have found that EFA metabolism may be abnormal in people with eczema. Supplementing with linoleic acid (omega-6 fatty acid), gamma-linolenic acid (found in borage oil), and evening primrose oil have all been explored in the treatment of eczema.[82]

My Recommendations

Children with allergies, asthma, and eczema may benefit from taking a daily vitamin and mineral supplementation. This should be a combination of vitamins and minerals. Two important components the supplement regimen should include are vitamin C and grape seed extract (a bioflavonoid). Also, increase their intake of omega-3 fats with the addition of omega-3 foods and an EFA supplement. CAUTION: High doses of omega-3 supplements may cause a slight *decline* in lung capacity in some asthmatics. Always consult your child's physician before starting a supplementation program.

In addition, environmental measures are very important in helping the child with asthma and allergies. Think of allergies like a bucket and when the bucket is full and overflowing, symptoms appear. There are things in the bucket that you can control like dust, mold, animal dander, and smoke. The more you can do to control these factors, the emptier the bucket will be, and there will be more room for things that you cannot control, like air pollution and pollens. (See below for measures to improve the environment of the child with allergies and asthma.)

Environmental Measures for the Child with Allergies, Asthma, and Eczema

- Dust and vacuum frequently in the child's bedroom.

- Use a microfilter vacuum bag that traps small dust particles better than a regular vacuum bag or consider buying a HEPA filter vacuum.

- Remove stuffed animals from the bedroom, even if they are on the shelves. They harbor dust mites.

- Use a dust-proof mattress pad for the mattress and box springs. These totally encase the mattress. Dust-proof pillow covers should also be used.

- Do not use down or feather comforters or pillows.

- Consider purchasing a HEPA air filter to run in the child's bedroom.

- Avoid second-hand smoke exposure for the child; you should especially avoid smoking in the car. Even if you smoke when the child is not present, smoke lingers.

- Consider taking the child off milk and soy products. Under a year of age, special hypoallergenic formulas can be tried *(Alimentum or Nutramigen)*. Over one year of age, rice milk may be used. Between a year and two years of age, rice milk is too low in fat, so supplement with essential fatty acids.

- If you have pets, do not allow them in the child's bedroom. Consider having allergy testing for animals if your child has significant symptoms, and you have pets. It may be time to get rid of them.

- Talk to your physician about allergy testing with blood work or doing scratch tests with an allergist if your child is miserable with allergies or asthma most of the time.

- Consider using an artificial Christmas tree or limiting the time the tree is in the house if you notice worsening of symptoms with the tree in the house.

- Watch for and remove mold growth in bathrooms and on windows (especially if you use a humidifier in the child's room).

- In addition, for eczema:

  - keep the skin moisturized (*Triceram* is a new lipid moisturizer that I have seen excellent results with eczema patients. See Appendix V for ordering information.)

  - avoid wool, nylon, or stiff materials that don't "breathe"

  - look for food allergies. (See p. 74, "Facts on Food Allergies.")

  - use tepid, not hot water for baths and keep them short

  - control dust in the environment.

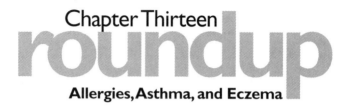

Chapter Thirteen

roundup

Allergies, Asthma, and Eczema

- Use a program of antioxidants, bioflavonoids, and essential fatty acids and monitor improvement. Doses may need to be adjusted, depending on the child, how significant the symptoms are, and the time of year that affects the child.

- Try to reduce environmental allergens like dust and mold and avoid second-hand smoke exposure. Consider pet exposures as a source of allergens and have your child tested if you are concerned about animal allergies.

- Carefully observe the times when your child has symptoms and try to identify triggers.

- Look at your child's misery level when deciding if you need to add or adjust pharmaceutical (prescription) drugs.

CAUTION: Consult your child's physician before starting a nutritional supplementation program.

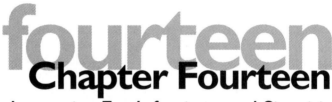

Chapter Fourteen
Immunity: Ear Infections and Sinusitis

Parents come into my office wondering why so many more children are suffering from ear infections and sinusitis than when they were growing up. Is it the environment, daycare, or over-treatment on the part of doctors? It may be a combination of all of these things. The environment has been implicated in increasing the rates of allergies and asthma; children with allergies often have an increased risk of infections. With more children going to daycare, these children are exposed to a greater number of colds and viruses that may lead to ear infections.

Doctors have been faulted in the past with over diagnosing ear infections and readily prescribing antibiotics for mild types of infections that may resolve on their own. The medical community is concerned that bacteria are developing resistance to antibiotics. There has been a change in parents' expectations of the doctor visit. Ten years ago, parents were often disappointed if their child did not receive antibiotics after an office visit. Today, more parents want to be sure their child really needs antibiotics when they are prescribed and rightly so. Doctors are also being encouraged to shift the way they practice and prescribe fewer antibiotics. Some ear infections are now observed without antibiotic treatment if the child does not appear ill and if the ear has fluid behind it without signs of a raging infection.

Micronutrients and Immunity

Can bad diets and nutrient deficiencies breed deadlier viruses and stress the immune system? Some highlights of the research in this area include:

- In developing countries, vitamin A deficiency is a public health problem. In a study from Turkey, serum vitamin A and beta-carotene levels were lower in children with recurrent acute respiratory infections than those children who were healthy.[83] In South Africa, children with lower vitamin A levels had more severe acute respiratory infections.[84]

- In a study in developing countries (where children are undernourished and often zinc deficient), zinc supplements were given to children. They found that the number of respiratory infections decreased by more than 40 percent. Pneumonia and other lower respiratory infections cause some four million deaths per year and make up one-third of all deaths among children in developing countries. Poor nutrition can increase the rate of these infections and their severity.[85] The incidence of diarrhea infections was also reduced in children supplemented with zinc in developing countries who were at risk for zinc deficiency.[86]

- The effect of zinc lozenges has shown mixed evidence of benefiting the common cold. One review of seven randomized controlled trials concluded that zinc did reduce the symptoms and duration of colds. However, the lozenges had to be taken every two hours and compliance with this regimen is a problem.[87] Another randomized controlled trial showed that zinc lozenges were not effective in treating cold symptoms in children and adolescents.[88] We may see that for children at risk for zinc deficiency (especially for those children in developing countries), more benefits may be likely, than those without a zinc deficiency.

- Vitamin C supplementation for colds has also met with mixed reviews. One interesting review of vitamin C supplementation showed that subjects under heavy physical stress did have benefits with vitamin C supplementation. There was a reduction in the number of colds in three groups undergoing intense physical activity: school children at a ski camp in the Swiss Alps, military troops training in Northern Canada, and participants in a 90 km running race.[89]

- People with chronic sinusitis have decreased amounts of two out of three important antioxidant substances when tested in the tissue of the nose as compared to healthy people.[90]

- Studies are reporting that children who chew gum or swallow a syrup containing *xylitol*, a sweetener, experience significantly fewer ear infections. The incidence of ear infections was reduced by 30 percent in one study.[91] Xylitol has been found to decrease the incidence of dental cavities, presumably, by inhibiting the growth of certain bacteria in the mouth.

- Selenium is a cofactor that works with vitamin E. It is found in meats and grains, but is dependent on the soil content where the food was raised. China, New Zealand, and certain areas of the United States have low selenium in the soils. Research is appearing on how selenium deficiency may trigger viral mutations creating more dangerous forms of the virus. Coxsackie viruses, which are a group of common viruses, are generally considered benign. It can cause fever and blisters in the mouth, called hand-foot-and-mouth disease.

In China, a deadly disease called Keshan disease (a cardiomyopathy, which is a form of heart failure of the muscle) has been associated with selenium deficiency. Researchers have discovered that coxsackie virus is the trigger for this disease and they postulate that selenium deficiency weakens the immunity and allows the virus to mutate to a more serious form.

• Another serious complication of poor nutrition is research that shows that deficiencies of selenium allowed viruses, like the influenza virus to mutate to more virulent forms. These forms are more aggressive and these mutations of new viral strains may make it even a more serious virus for someone with normal nutritional status.[92]

• Drug-induced nutrient depletion is an under recognized problem. Most physicians understand that diuretics used for fluid overload in cardiac adult patients can cause potassium depletion. However, antibiotics like penicillins, cephalosporins, and sulfonamides have been found to deplete the B vitamins. Ibuprofen causes a depletion of folic acid. With the number of antibiotics many children are on, it seems wise to cover for this array of nutrient deficiencies.[93]

Acute Otitis Media (Middle Ear Infection)

Acute otitis media occurs when infected fluid is found in the middle ear space, which is the space behind the eardrum. The eardrum appears red and swollen, and yellow pus can be seen in the middle ear space. This type of infection usually accompanies a cold. This is typically painful, although this pain can vary. It is most common in children between six months and three or four years of age. Earwax, water, or wind in the ear does not cause middle ear infections. Water in the ear can cause a different problem called *swimmer's ear (otitis externa)*, which is an infection of the skin in the ear canal.

Sometimes there is fluid behind the eardrum that is not infected, called *otitis media with effusion* or *serous otitis media*. This commonly occurs after an acute ear infection has been treated. The child is not in pain or ill-appearing, and the eardrum is not red or inflamed. This does not necessarily need to be treated with antibiotics. This fluid may be present for weeks to months.

What are the signs of an acute ear infection?

Listed below are common symptoms of an acute ear infection. However, some children have no real symptoms other than they are not "acting right." The only way to diagnose ear infections is to have a physician look in the ear.

• Fussy babies, cranky toddlers

• Babies may pull off the bottle or breast several times and cry

• Not sleeping well

- Usually accompany a cold
- May or may not have a fever
- Pulling on the ear (pulling on the ear in a happy, non-sick child may be a sign of teething)
- Fluid (blood or pus) draining from the ear
- Not hearing well, talking loudly, ignoring normal voice tones, television volume increased
- Older child complaining of pain.

> Check out **www.callyourped.com**
> to learn more about common childhood illnesses

What are factors that can contribute to ear infections?

- **Large adenoids.** Children who snore and open-mouth breathe may have large adenoids, and these can impinge on the *Eustachian tube*. (This is the tube that drains the middle ear to the nasal passage; the tube we "pop" when we fly.) Large adenoids block drainage from the middle ear and allow fluid to build up and stay in the middle ear. The adenoids cannot be seen except on a lateral neck X-ray or with special equipment by an ear, nose, and throat specialist.

- **Daycare settings.** Ear infections are not contagious, but the virus that started the cold is contagious. Children in daycare will average one cold a month in the winter months, and for some children, every cold seems to turn into an ear infection.

- **Taking a bottle or breastfeeding lying down.** Lying down and sucking on the bottle or breast can cause some aspiration of liquid through the Eustachian tube and into the middle ear. Pacifier use may also increase the risk of ear infections.

- **Allergies.** Constant nasal stuffiness can block the Eustachian tube and lead to ear infections.

- **Spitting up.** A baby who spits up a lot may be at more risk for ear infections.

- **Second-hand smoke.** Smoking environments raise the risks of developing ear infections and may prolong the recovery from ear infections.

- **Water going up the nose.** Swimming under water or diving in the water pushes water up the nose, back up through the Eustachian tube, and into the middle ear.

- **Flying with a cold.** Children who take plane flights with a cold have trouble equalizing their middle ear pressure and this may lead to an ear infection.

- **Family history.** If parents had a history of a lot of ear infections, their children may be prone to the same problem.

Sinusitis

Sinusitis is an infection of the sinus spaces, which are small air-filled spaces around the structure of the nasal passage. This is caused by a bacterial infection. Sometimes, ear infections and sinus infections occur together. Signs of sinusitis include:

- Runny nose or congestion more than 10 to 14 days, especially if getting worse
- Clear, green, or yellow mucous may be present (colored mucous does not always mean a sinus infection)
- Decreased appetite
- Crankiness
- Cough, especially at night or in the morning
- Headaches or tenderness over the sinuses for older children
- A fever, in some, but not all cases.

Preventative Measures

If your child is getting recurrent or persistent ear infections, some issues should be examined to see if the situation can be improved. *Recurrent* means getting an ear infection within a few weeks of clearing a previous ear infection. *Persistent* means an ear that appears to have continued fluid behind it.

- Consider changing daycare to a smaller daycare or finding a sitter to come to the house. The more children a child is exposed to, the more risk for colds and then ear infections. In the daycare, try to find situations where there are not a lot of drop-in children. Drop-in daycares, for example at the local gym, are a problem because there are different children around at every visit, and there are many children visiting within a day. The daycare setting is especially important with young babies under a year or two.
- Never give a bottle or breastfeed a baby lying down.
- Avoid second-hand smoke.
- Search for possible allergies. If your child seems congested most of the time and other family members or daycare members are not getting sick, allergies may be a possibility. A trial off all dairy and soy products may be helpful. (See p. 74, "Facts on Food Allergies," and Chapter 13.)
- Spitting up excessively may lead to ear infections in infants. Measures like burping frequently and keeping the baby's head elevated 20 minutes after feeding may be helpful. Medications to treat spitting up are sometimes needed and this should be discussed with your doctor. (See p. 78, "Spitting Up.")
- Avoid swimming with the head under water or diving and jumping in the water, especially if a cold is present. Swimming under water tends to push water up the nose and may cause reflux of fluid into the Eustachian tube that may lead to an ear infection.

Medical Treatment for Recurrent or Persistent Ear Infections

- **Antibiotics.** These are used to treat acute ear infections. If your child does need to be on antibiotics, *Lactobacillus acidophilus* and *Lactobacillus bifidus* may be beneficial in combating yeast. It is best to use a supplement that can be found at health food stores. A study from Finland showed that children in daycare who took *Lactobacillus* had less respiratory and intestinal infections.[94]

- **Low dose preventative antibiotics.** Low doses of a daily antibiotic for a month or two may prevent infections from recurring. Antibiotics may be used for a child who just has fluid behind the ear that does not appear infected to prevent it from becoming infected. Although we are concerned about antibiotic overuse, a low dose of one antibiotic over a period of time is probably better for a child's system than using three or four different antibiotics over the same period of time.

- **Tubes in the ears.** Tiny plastic tubes are placed surgically into the eardrum by an ear, nose, and throat surgeon to allow ventilation and drainage from the middle ear to the outside. This option is often considered if a child has had about three months of a chronic ear infection or continues to have recurrent ear infection despite low dose antibiotics.

- **Removing adenoids.** Large adenoids are often suspected if your child snores at night and open-mouth breathes in the day. These can increase the risks for middle ear infections. Removing the adenoids may be beneficial with or without placement of ear tubes at the same time.

Chapter Fourteen
roundup
Immunity: Ear Infections and Sinusitis

- Pursue the preventative measures listed in this chapter.

- If you suspect allergies are playing a role in your child's ear infections, review the previous chapter on allergies and asthma.

- Use a supplement that has vitamin C, zinc, and beta-carotene.

- Bioflavonoids, as found in grape seed extract, may be helpful. It has anti-inflammatory effects and may benefit the child who gets recurrent ear infections.

- Try xylitol gum for the older child or look for a children's vitamin sweetened with xylitol (see Appendix V).

CAUTION: Consult your child's physician before starting a nutritional supplementation program.

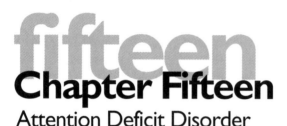

Chapter Fifteen
Attention Deficit Disorder

Attention deficit disorder (ADD), or hyperactivity as it was called in the past, is a disorder that seems to be diagnosed more often. From 1990 to 1995, there was a 2.5-fold increase in the use of methylphenidate (*Ritalin*), a popular drug used to treat ADD in children 5 to 18 years of age.[95] In 1998, it has been estimated that 3 to 5 percent of school-aged children (2.5 to 3 million children) have ADD.

What is ADD?

Most parents have probably had thoughts at one time or another about their child having this problem. Health professionals rarely diagnose ADD before the age of four years. There is not a single laboratory or standardized test that can be definitively used to diagnose ADD. It is diagnosed based on a clinical picture of behaviors. This information must be collected by interviews or questionnaires with parents, teachers, caretakers, and the child. There are various behavior rating scales and cognitive tests that are used to help make the diagnosis. Because these tests are subjective, it is sometimes difficult to be certain of the diagnosis. There may be other problems occurring along with the ADD that may make it difficult to sort out. Learning disabilities, depression, oppositional behavior, and family problems may occur with ADD or may be the underlying problem causing their behavior. ADD is a syndrome that is characterized with difficulties resulting in poor attention span, lack of impulse control and/or hyperactivity. Some common symptoms can include:

- fails to give close attention to details or makes careless mistakes in schoolwork, work, or other activities

- has difficulty sustaining attention in tasks or play activities and is easily distracted by extraneous stimuli

- does not follow through on instructions and fails to finish schoolwork, chores, or duties in the workplace (not due to oppositional behavior or failure to understand instructions)

- is forgetful in daily activities

- fidgets with hands or feet or squirms in seat or runs about or climbs excessively

- talks excessively or blurts out answers before questions have been completed

- has difficulty awaiting turn

What Causes ADD?

A single cause of ADD has not been scientifically proven. It is most likely to be a result of several different factors. Some possible causes that have been explored:

- **Genetic/hereditary.** ADD has a genetic basis. Adoption studies have shown more of a genetic rather than environmental influence.

- **Brain damage by toxins.** Children born with fetal alcohol syndrome have been found to have a higher rate of ADD. Lead poisoning, pesticide exposure (see Chapter 2), and traumatic or infectious injury to the brain may lead to increased activity and poor attention span.

- **Food allergies and sensitivity to sugar and/or additives.** This is a controversial area of treating ADD. In his 1975 book, *Why Your Child is Hyperactive*, Dr. Ben Feingold hypothesized that salicylates, aspirin-like substances in foods, and artificial dyes and colors were the cause of hyperactivity in children. (Salicylates in foods are found in almonds and other nuts, apples, citrus fruits, and dried fruits. Many food additives and artificial food colors and preservatives, like BHT, are salicylates.) Feingold's book was based purely on clinical experience, and since then, the medical community has been trying to support or refute his theory. Studies have shown mixed results, some concluding no difference with diet changes, and some studies showing improvement in behavior.

- **Visual problems.** Occasionally, a child with a visual tracking problem may appear to have ADD, but merely have a visual problem called *"convergence insufficiency."* These children will have poor reading skills, but usually maintain high math problem-solving skills. If you suspect this, a complete eye exam is recommended.

- **Other risk factors.** Relationships with a low-birth-weight, prolonged labor, and poor social status have been found. Boys with ADD outnumber girls by three to one.

Environmental Causes of ADD

Research is ongoing to find a cause of ADD. The role of environmental toxins and pollutants is one area of research. Studies are typically performed on animals, and it is difficult to prove if this translates to the human model. However, in light of some of the research provided below, it may be important for a pregnant mother and young children to try to limit exposure to environmental toxins.

- Fetal exposure to environmental pollutants such as dioxins and polychlorinated biphenyls (PCBs) may impede neurological development, lower adult IQ, and increase the risk for attention deficit hyperactivity disorder. Mass poisonings that occurred in Japan in 1968 and in Taiwan in 1979 were the basis of gathering this information.[96]

- A study done in a community in Sonora, Mexico, looked at two populations of children, ages four to five, in the area. The first group living in the valley, were exposed to heavy pesticides from their farming community, and received exposure to household bug sprays. They had detectable concentrations of many pesticides in their blood. The second group in the foothills had little pesticide exposure and did not use household bug spray. The children in the first group showed less stamina and had poor performance on gross and fine motor coordination, 30-minute recall, and drawing ability.[97]

Key nutrients during pregnancy and after birth have been examined as playing a possible role in brain development.

- Choline, a B-complex vitamin, plays a role in cognitive development both prior to and after birth. For this reason the National Academy of Sciences has recommended pregnant women take 450 mg per day and nursing women take 550 mg per day of choline. In a study, pregnant rats were fed no choline, limited amounts, or high doses of choline. Pups born to mothers that received no choline did poorly on tests designed to measure attention and certain types of memory. The behavioral effects of choline availability in utero were long-lasting and persisted beyond the age of two years, this is an age when a rat is considered developmentally old.[98]

- Essential fatty acids are important for development of infant cognitive behavior and brain development. Whether a lack of EFA during pregnancy or birth may have a role in attention deficit disorder needs to be studied. In the discussion below, research has shown that some children with ADD have lower essential fatty acid levels.

The Role of Diet and Micronutrients on ADD

There has been much interest about diet and micronutrients in the treatment of ADD. Evidence in the medical literature shows mixed results. Initial studies in the 1970's and early 1980's showed more often that the relationship between diet and hyperactivity was not valid, however, researchers of the late 1980's and the 1990's showed a possible relationship between the two. One of the problems with some of the earlier studies was that only a single elimination of a substance was performed. Later studies, which eliminated multiple items in their testing, seemed to reveal benefits to the elimination diet. However, these elimination diets are difficult to enforce in children.

The question of how sugar affects behavior has been one filled with different opinions. With my own son and his friends, I often observe the high energy behavior after a party filled with sugar and sweets. However, I have also seen energy surges after normal meals without sweets. One theory is that high glycemic index foods. (See p. 150, "Glycemic Index.") might be a contributing factor to behavior problems. These foods cause a rapid spike in glucose and insulin and may create the "sugar rush" that people can experience. You may want to try low glycemic foods and see how it affects your child's behavior.

The following highlights some of the more recent studies linking diet and nutrients to ADD:

- In a 1988 study of 220 children with "hyperactivity," 55 were placed on a six-week trial of the Feingold diet. Forty (72.7 percent) showed improved behavior and 26 (47.3 percent) remained improved following liberalization of the diet over a period of 3 to 6 months.[99]

- A diet that eliminated artificial colors, flavors, chocolate, monosodium glutamate, preservatives, and caffeine was tested in 24 hyperactive preschool boys in a 1989 study. The diet was also low in sugar and dairy free if the family reported a history of possible problems with these foods. There was improvement in behavior in 58 percent of children.[100]

- An analysis was done of all the studies on the effects of sugar and behavior from 1984 to 1994. Statistical analysis found that sugar does not affect the behavior or cognitive performance of children. However, the researchers that "the current number of studies doesn't eliminate the possibility of a small effect." They also found that results where the parents rated behavior changes due to sugar intake were more likely to show positive benefits of eliminating sugar than if an independent researcher rated behavior. This is most likely because of parents' expectations of how sugar may affect their child.[101]

- A simple diet elimination of sugar or candy was not convincing in a repeated placebo-controlled challenge study in 1996.[102]

- In a study reported in 1994 in the *Annals of Allergy*, 26 children with ADD had a diet that eliminated multiple items, including dairy, wheat, corn, yeast, soy, citrus, egg, chocolate, peanuts, artificial colors, and preservatives for two weeks. Nineteen children (73 percent) showed improvement on this diet. Food challenges were performed on those children who responded to the elimination diet over the next month as a double-blind placebo-controlled trial by masking the foods or dyes. All of the children reacted with increased activity to three or more items. In this study, most of the children who responded to diet changes tended to be children who also had allergy problems, like asthma, eczema, and allergic rhinitis.[103]

- Seventy-eight children with hyperactive behavior were placed on a restricted diet that only allowed a few foods (meats, rice and potatoes, and two fruits, green and root vegetables, milk-free margarine, bottled water, and sunflower oil) in this 1993 study. Fifty-nine had improved behavior. For 19 of these children, foods and additives were disguised with other foods in a placebo-controlled double-blind challenge. Results here showed a significant effect for the provoking foods to worsen ratings of behavior.[104]

The conclusions that come to light about diet and behavior in ADD children are that a small group of children may respond to diet elimination. Subjects who show more allergic tendencies seem to be better responders to dietary changes and elimination of allergenic type foods. The main challenge is to define which type of children will be diet responders. Some of the more common foods implicated in causing ADD symptoms from some of these studies include artificial colors and preservatives, soy milk, soybeans, soy sauce, cow's milk, chocolate, grapes, wheat, oranges, eggs, peanuts, corn, fish, oats, melon, and tomato.[105]

Nutritional Supplementation

Nutritional supplementation with essential fatty acids, vitamins, and minerals has been studied. The essential fatty acids are important components of the neuronal cells of the brain. (See p. 55, "Fats: The Good, the Bad, and the Ugly.") Some results of these studies are presented below.

- Fifty-three children with ADD were noted to have significantly lower concentrations of fatty acids in their blood and within their red blood cells. Also, a subgroup of 21 patients with ADD had symptoms of essential fatty acid (EFA) deficiency and had much lower concentrations of certain fatty acid groups than those with ADD and few EFA deficiency symptoms. Symptoms of EFA deficiency include thirst, frequent urination, dry skin, dry hair, dandruff, and brittle nails.[106]

- Forty-eight children with ADD were evaluated and zinc and serum free fatty acid levels were significantly lower than those of controls.[107]

- The role of multivitamin preparations has suggested that mild deficiencies in diet and blood levels need to be investigated further. In 1991, in a double-blind placebo-controlled trial of RDA vitamin and mineral supplementation in 47 six-year-olds not selected for ADD, researchers found an improvement in IQ (8.3 points), an increase in concentration, a decrease in fidgeting on a frustrating task, and an advantage on a reaction time task assessing sustained attention. Trials with megavitamin cocktails and megadoses of specific vitamins have not shown success.[108] [109]

- Iron supplementation has been found to cause some improvement in ADD children. Researchers studied non-anemic boys with ADD and supplemented them with iron. They had improvement in parents' ratings of behavior, but not in teachers' ratings.[110] Another study showed improved verbal learning and memory in a double-blind placebo-controlled trial of teenage non-anemic, but iron-deficient girls (mild iron deficiency can be present without having significant anemia).[111]

- Zinc may have a role in ADD children. Zinc deficiency is known to impair concentration and cause jitteriness. Animal studies have found a role of zinc deficiency in hyperactivity. Zinc has been reported to be lower in ADD children when compared with controls.[112]

- Magnesium deficiency was noted in 95 percent of a group of 116 children with ADD. When 50 of these magnesium deficient children were supplemented with magnesium and compared to controls, the supplemented group had improvement in behavior.[113]

- Jean Carper, in her book *Miracle Cures*, discusses the benefits of using grape seed extract in patients with ADD. Some patients had noted improvement in attention and concentration with grape seed extract. It has been found in cell culture studies that it may affect brain cells by helping control two neurotransmitters, dopamine and norepinephrine. Grape seed extract may also help in the transfer of minerals, like zinc, manganese, selenium, and copper to the brain.[114]

Treatment of ADD

To cover the various aspects of ADD treatment is beyond the scope of this book. However, I will summarize the well-recognized treatments, and talk about some of the controversial aspects of treatment that are available. ADD requires a multiple-modality approach. This combines psychosocial interventions as well as medical interventions. Children with ADD do not respond to the usual behavior management techniques. Parent training is an important aspect of managing a child with ADD. Schools and teachers must be willing to work with these children and recognize that these children may need to be handled differently. A structured classroom with the child seated in the front row allows the child to focus more readily. While most children can remain in a regular classroom setting, some may need extra tutoring. Some with more complex problems may need a special class or a special school directed to children with learning and behavior problems. Child-focused intervention may include psychotherapy to deal with issues of·low self-esteem, anxiety, or depression, and to help the child improve social skills and impulse control. Finding community support groups that allow you to connect with other families with children with ADD is helpful. (See Appendix VII for resources.)

The use of medications has long been the mainstay treatment of ADD. However, some people have concerns that we are overmedicating our young. Sometimes teachers refer children who have difficult behavior problems, not necessarily ADD, for treatment with medications. As a parent, it is often a difficult and grueling decision when deciding to medicate. However, the benefits for those children who need medications can be remarkable. My advice to parents is to make sure you have had a thorough evaluation and are comfortable with the information you are receiving. Seek second opinions if necessary. To most parents of children with ADD, it is obvious that they are dealing with children who have extra challenges. To see improved behavior and improved learning potential with appropriate treatment can be a relief.

Dietary intervention is becoming more accepted in the medical community as playing a role in treatment of ADD. Here are my suggestions for diet and nutritional supplementation in children with ADD.

- **Don't count on dietary changes or nutritional supplementation to treat or cure ADD.** Some benefits may appear, but many children will still need other treatments like behavior modification and/or medication. Do not stop prescribed medications without consulting your health professional. It is best to try dietary intervention first and discuss reducing doses of medications if the child appears to show improvement. If you have "drug-free" periods on weekends or vacations, take particular note of behavior changes if you are working on dietary intervention.

- **Look for signs of allergies.** If your child has been diagnosed with allergic rhinitis, asthma, or eczema, a trial period without the more common allergenic foods may be beneficial. An excellent book that covers the role of allergies in behavior and how to identify these is by Dr. Doris Rapp, entitled *Is This Your Child?*

- **Try an elimination diet.** This may be a difficult task for most families and should be undertaken with the approval of your child's pediatrician. A simple place to start is by eliminating dairy, wheat, eggs, and nuts for three to four weeks. You may re-challenge one food group at a time after the elimination and observe behavior. A stricter approach would be to eliminate artificial colors, flavors, preservatives, cow's milk, cheese, yogurt, chocolate, and caffeine drinks. Try choosing low glycemic foods and avoid the high glycemic foods, such as sugar, white bread, and processed carbohydrates (crackers, cereals, bagels, and chips).

- **Try using a balanced combination of vitamins and minerals.** Zinc, copper, manganese, and selenium should be included in the supplement.

- **Add essential fatty acids foods and supplements.** Dosages have not been defined. Try to include more canola oil, flaxseed oil, and fatty fish, like salmon, fresh tuna, sardines, and mackerel. Consider adding an essential fatty acid supplement. (See p. 59, "Essential Fatty Acids: Benefits and Sources.")

- **Look for signs of essential fatty acid deficiency.** These include excess thirst, frequent urination, dry hair, dry skin, dandruff, and small hard flesh-colored bumps (called keratosis piliaris) on the arms and thighs. (NOTE: Excess thirst and frequent urination may be a sign of diabetes. If you see these symptoms, a urine test should be done to look for glucose in the urine.) If you notice signs of EFA deficiency, see if, after a month of supplementation, the symptoms disappear and if behavior improves.

- **Add grape seed extract.** Dosages have not been well studied. Start with 60 to 90 mg of grape seed extract a day for a week for a school age child and increase this by 15 to 30 mg per week. Higher doses of grape seed extract may cause diarrhea, but otherwise have not been found to have other side effects.

Chapter Fifteen
roundup
Attention Deficit Disorder

- Treatment of attention deficit disorder is a complex problem, and requires a multi-disciplinary approach.

- The diet can be changed and nutritional supplementation can be added. Some children may see some benefits.

- Use a vitamin and mineral supplement, an omega-3 supplement, and grape seed extract. (See Appendix VI.)

- Consultation with a health professional who deals with ADD children and being communicative with the school are two necessary parts of treating ADD.

- Be supportive and do your own research.

CAUTION: Consult your child's physician before starting a nutritional supplementation program.

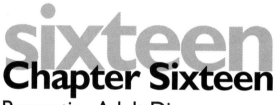

Chapter Sixteen
Preventing Adult Diseases
Now and in the Future

Why include a discussion of adult diseases in a book about children's health and nutrition? The first reason is because our children are future adults. What they are eating today will create certain risks for diseases as they age. It may be years until we understand long-term issues, like could a child who is given vitamin E supplements reduce their risks of Alzheimer's disease or heart disease as an adult? Secondly, we are seeing more adolescents and young adults developing diseases that were traditionally thought to be diseases of old age. Diseases like hypertension and adult-onset diabetes are occurring in younger age groups.

The last reason to include this chapter is because you, the reader, are most likely a parent and an adult. If you are really interested in teaching your child healthy eating habits, you must be the role model. It is a big responsibility that must be taken seriously. It will be nearly impossible for your child to eat healthy if you are frequently eating fast foods, high-fat, sugary desserts, or high-fat snacks. If I can convince you of the benefits of healthy eating and nutritional supplementation, you will be more convinced to do this for yourself and for your family.

Cardiovascular Disease

Heart disease is the number one killer, and stroke is the number three killer in the United States today. Statistics for the United States reveal:

- Two out of five Americans will eventually die of heart disease
- Deaths annually from heart disease: 733,834
- Deaths annually from stroke: 160,431
- Cases reported annually of heart disease: 22.3 million
- Cases reported annually of stroke: 3 million

Despite all the modern advances in medicine, there is not a "cure" for heart disease and stroke. There are hundreds of pharmaceutical drugs designed to reduce chest pain, improve heart function, lower blood pressure, and thin the blood to reduce the risks of clots occurring in the blood vessels of the heart. Prevention is key to reducing the rates of cardiovascular disease. Lifestyle and diet can dramatically reduce the risks of cardiovascular disease. Obesity increases the risk for high cholesterol and hypertension, which are two other risk factors for heart disease and stroke.

In addition, a new link to the development of atherosclerosis (the hardening of the arteries that leads to heart attack and stroke) is *homocysteine*. This is an amino acid that is a by-product of our normal metabolism. High levels of homocysteine have been found to increase the risk for atherosclerosis. It is now proposed in research studies that homocysteine damages arterial walls and promotes the deposition of fatty plaques, which leads to atherosclerosis. Due to environmental or genetic factors, a person may have a tendency to have higher levels of homocysteine. Medical research is accumulating on the role of vitamin B-6, vitamin B-12, and folate in lowering homocysteine levels. People with the highest levels of B-6, B-12, and folate in their blood have the lowest risk of heart disease.

Atherosclerosis can appear in the arteries in those as young as age 15.[115] Targeting our children and adolescents is the key to primary prevention efforts against heart attacks and strokes. Following are some of the studies that look at the pediatric population and their risks for future cardiovascular disease, as referred to earlier in Chapter 3:

- A study in the *Journal of the American Medical Association,* April 1999, looked at children in the eighth-grade and measured their homocysteine levels. This is the first large U.S. study to measure homocysteine in children. Children who did not take a multivitamin had 6 percent more homocysteine than children who took even one vitamin a week. The children who took daily vitamins were the most protected from high homocysteine levels. Currently, this evidence does not mean that vitamins for children will prevent heart attacks or strokes later in life, but we certainly need to study this issue further.[116]

- Overweight children were more likely to have high blood pressure and high cholesterol, especially of the low-density lipoprotein, which is the "bad" cholesterol. These factors could increase their risk for cardiovascular disease later in life.[117]

- An eight-week study of over 2,000 third and fourth graders showed that a simple educational program aimed at reducing heart risk factors could cut cholesterol and body fat in as little as eight weeks. Children were divided into three groups. The first group was instructed by their classroom teacher on the importance of exercise and how to select heart-healthy foods. They also did aerobic exercises three times per week. In the second group, children identified at risk for cardiovascular disease were separated from classmates, were taught the same aerobic exercises, and were told about good nutrition. The third group received no special instruction. After eight weeks, the first two groups that received heart-health instruction showed large drops in cholesterol compared to the control group. The instructed children also had a small reduction in body fat and higher health knowledge.[118]

Adult medical literature is filled with studies on the benefits to the cardiovascular system from various antioxidants and minerals. A few relevant clinical studies are summarized here:

- For 750 patients who placed in the bottom 20 percent of the group in terms of blood levels of vitamin B-6, they doubled their risk of heart disease over those patients with the highest levels of B-6. Similarly, low levels of folic acid were associated with an increased risk of vascular disease.[119]

- A review of 27 previously published studies on homocysteine concluded that a high level of homocysteine was a risk factor for vascular disease. The majority of patients with elevated homocysteine were deficient in folic acid, vitamin B-6, and vitamin B-12.[120]

- In a study of 2,002 patients with proven heart disease, vitamin E supplements reduced non-fatal heart attacks by 77 percent.[121]

- Among patients who had coronary atherosclerosis, low blood levels of vitamin C were associated with recurring chest pain or a heart attack.[122]

- Fish oil supplements were found to decrease the mortality risk in patients who already had a heart attack. Dr. Gianni Tognoni and colleagues across Italy studied over 11,500 heart attack patients and found that taking fish oil supplements reduced their risk of dying from heart disease by 15 percent.[123]

- Patients with cardiomyopathy (a weakening of the heart muscle) and congestive heart failure who received coenzyme Q10 supplementation had improved cardiac function.[124]

Because research on the role of supplements for decreasing risks of cardiovascular disease is primarily done on adults, researchers need to evaluate the value of supplements for our children to decrease these same risks. This will take many more years. Do our children have time to wait, or should we be considering supplements now? Our children's heart-health risks are high. They have more exposure to processed, fatty foods than any other generation to date. Consider the evidence and the risks for not doing anything. Adults and children need to eat a healthy diet, exercise, and use a nutritional supplement to decrease risks of cardiovascular disease.

Cancer

Today, cancer is the second leading cause of death behind cardiovascular disease in the United States. There is concern that cancer may overtake heart disease as the number one killer. After adjusting for factors like longevity, it has been shown that there are considerably more cancer deaths now than there were among Americans born between 1888 through 1897.[125] Experts have proven links between diet, obesity, and environmental factors for different types of cancer. We know smoking increases the risk of lung cancer, eating red meat increases the risk of colon cancer, chewing tobacco increases the risk of oral cancer, and sun exposure increases the risk of skin cancer. Every day we read in newspapers about a new carcinogen. Carcinogens increase free radical production, and when these free radicals bombard the DNA of the cell, the cell may undergo changes that allow a mutation. The cell will replicate out of control, and then the cancer will become clinically evident. The evidence is overwhelming that eating fruits and vegetables with their variety of antioxidants is a powerful defense against cancer. For those patients diagnosed with cancer, dietary intervention is entering mainstream treatment for the disease.

A ground-breaking study that opened the eyes of the medical community appeared in the *Journal of the American Medical Association* in December 1996. In this double-blind, placebo-controlled study of over 1,000 patients, researchers found that patients who received supplementation with 200 micrograms of selenium had a

- 37 percent decrease in cancer incidence
- 50 percent decrease in cancer mortality
- 63 percent decrease in prostate cancer
- 46 percent decrease in lung cancer
- 58 percent decrease in colorectal cancer.[126]

Other studies related to cancer prevention:

- Long-term supplementation with a multivitamin with folate may reduce the risk of colon cancer in women by as much as 75 percent. Women who took more than 400 micrograms per day of folic acid were 31 percent less likely to develop colon cancer.[127]
- There was a large study done in China in an area that had a high rate of stomach and esophageal cancer. Patients with early cellular change of these types of cancer who supplemented with beta-carotene, vitamin E, and selenium showed a 13 percent reduction in cancer mortality and a 21 percent reduction in stomach cancer mortality.[128]

- High intakes of lutein, zeaxanthin, and beta-carotene from food and supplements protected premenopausal women from the risks of breast cancer.[129]

- Bioflavonoids have been shown to inhibit tumor growth in animals and slow the development of new blood vessels within the tumor.[130] Bioflavonoids are excellent scavengers of free radicals and are about 50 times more potent an antioxidant than vitamin E.

- A diet high in fiber (anywhere from 20 to 35 grams) can lower the risk of some cancers.

- A study in hamsters showed that a combination of antioxidants (beta-carotene, vitamin E, glutathione, and vitamin C) worked best together, rather than alone, to inhibit the growth of experimentally induced oral cancer. The power of the synergy of antioxidants was shown in this study.[131]

- A combination of antioxidants (vitamin C, vitamin E, and beta-carotene), essential fatty acids, and coenzyme Q10 was given to 32 high-risk breast cancer patients. Observations included:

    (1) None of the patients died (the expected number was 4)

    (2) None had further distant metastases

    (3) Quality of life improved (no weight loss, reduced pain killers)

    (4) Six patients showed apparent partial remission.[132]

Nutritional therapy in cancer patients needs more research. Based on research we have so far, there are some measures we can take that may decrease our cancer risk. Recommendations on how to decrease cancer risks are provided in the following chart.

Recommendations to Decrease Cancer Risks

- **Increase intake of fruits, vegetables, and whole grains.** Include lots of cruciferous vegetables (broccoli, cauliflower, cabbage, Brussels sprouts, and onions) and tomato products. (Tomatoes contain lycopene, which may decrease risks of prostate cancer.)

- **Eat a low-fat diet,** meaning less than 20 to 30 percent of total calories should be from fat. Focus on lowering saturated fats (saturated fats are found in butter, cream, milk, most pastries, and fatty portions of meats and chicken). Use more monosaturated (like olive oil, canola oils) and polyunsaturated fats (in vegetable and fish oils). Remember: children under the age of two should not be restricted with a low-fat diet.

- **Eat a high-fiber diet** (at least 20 to 35 grams per day for teens and adults). Fruits, vegetables, legumes, and whole grains are all fiber sources. To calculate your child's fiber needs: add your child's age plus 5. So, for an 8-year-old, daily fiber intake should be 8 + 5 = 13 grams. (See Appendix II, "High Fiber Foods.")

- **Minimize foods that are heavy in hormones and reduce pesticide exposure** by using more organic foods or by washing and peeling conventionally grown fruits and vegetables. Hormones are used in poultry and meats, and also are found in milk.

- **Take antioxidants** to further protect against free radical damage that may trigger a cancer to develop. Important micronutrients to include are vitamin C, vitamin E, folate, beta-carotene, selenium, coenzyme Q10, bioflavonoids, and essential fatty acids.

Nutrients Associated with Disease Prevention

This information is taken from the Council of Responsible Nutrition report, *Optimal Nutrition for Good Health: The Benefits of Nutritional Supplements.*[133]

Nutrient	Helps Protect Against	Protective Daily Intake
Calcium	Osteoporosis	1,000 to 1,500 mg
Vitamin D	Osteoporosis	400 to 800 IU
Folic acid	Birth defects	0.4 to 0.8 mg
Folic acid	Heart disease and stroke	0.4 to 0.8 mg
Vitamin E	Heart disease	100 to 400 IU
Multivitamins	Infectious disease	RDA or greater
Antioxidants	Cataracts	*
Lutein/Zeaxanthin	Macular degeneration	*
Vitamin C	Stomach cancer	250 mg or more
Selenium	Some cancers	200 mcg
Carotenoids	Some cancers	*
Dietary fiber	Some cancers	20 to 25 grams
Soluble fiber	Heart disease	6 grams
Omega-3 PUFAs	Heart disease	1 to 3 grams

* Protective intake not yet determined.

This is only the tip of the iceberg as far as the research found in medical literature. To understand more details of this research, read Dr. Ray Strand's *Bionutrition: Winning the War Within* and Dr. Kenneth Cooper's *Advanced Nutritional Therapies.* These books present compelling evidence for the role of nutritional supplementation.

Chapter Sixteen
roundup
Preventing Adult Diseases
Now and in the Furture

- Understand the risks of future diseases on your child. Heart disease is much easier to prevent than treat. Diet has been shown to have a significant impact on heart disease and cancer risks.

- Make changes in your family's nutrition program and include a comprehensive supplementation program.

- Increase your family's fiber intake.

CAUTION: Consult your child's physician before starting a nutritional supplementation program.

conclusion

Conclusion:
Positive Success Tips for Parents

What are the most important lessons you learned from reading this book? I hope that you can make the following promise to your children.

A Promise of Good Health to My Children

I will provide my children with a variety of the most nutritious foods available.

I will provide my children the opportunity to be active and exercise regularly.

I will provide my children the highest quality, guaranteed, pharmaceutical-grade nutritional supplements.

How we feed our kids today is so important for their future. Kids who learn to eat great at an early age are more likely to stay healthy and receive the long-term benefits of good health as they age. They are more likely to reduce their risk of obesity and their risk of many of the degenerative diseases of aging. We may also be able to improve their health today and long after we are gone.

Parenting our children is a balancing act. We balance love and discipline, we balance play time and work time, we balance teaching our children and learning from our children, and we balance healthy eating and not-so-healthy eating. You need a little of all these things in the right proportion. Not allowing children to explore choices, even unhealthy ones, is not necessarily good. They will discover these choices despite us. But if we nurture their palate at an early age to encourage more healthy foods and demonstrate these lessons ourselves, our children are more likely to follow suit.

You need to do some very important homework now that you have read this book. Examine your own personal eating and exercise habits and encourage other adults in your household to do the same. See if you can become a better role model. Besides your own health benefits, of which there are many, think about the example you are setting for your children and the health benefits for them. Any parent who has watched their child sleep understands the overwhelming love and the overwhelming desire to protect their child. You certainly do not want to imagine atherosclerosis or other devastating diseases developing within their bodies. Encouraging good eating habits in children must start with a family effort practicing good eating habits.

If you read this book and you have a newborn, you are fortunate. You can start implementing the ideas here and work on creating healthy eating habits for your infant from day one. On the other hand, no matter what the age of your children, you can still nurture them with good nutrition now and expect positive results.

If you read this book and you are feeling guilty because you see that you should be doing more to create healthy eating habits for your family, don't feel overwhelmed or discouraged. Don't expect change to happen overnight. Make one small change every day—give up fast foods, find a store that carries organic foods, declare a moratorium on hot dogs, limit television time, educate yourself more about nutrition, learn about environmental threats and how to protect your family, start an exercise regimen, start a nutritional supplementation program—but make a change. Then tomorrow it will be easier to make another change and then another. Move in a positive direction of leading a healthy lifestyle, and you will be giving your children a gift for a lifetime.

Let's teach our kids to eat great and love it!

APPENDIX

Growth
Charts

Girls: Birth to 36 Months

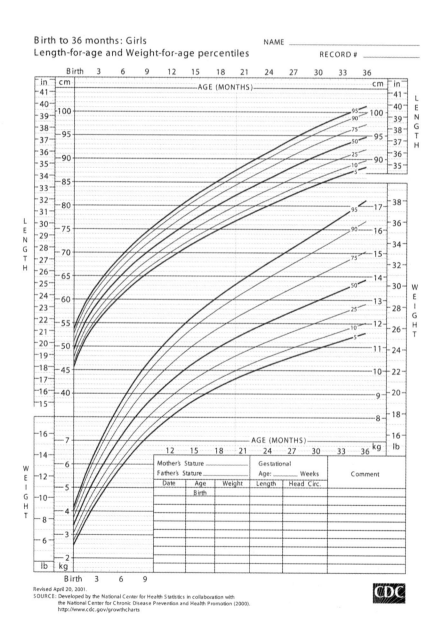

Birth to 36 months: Girls
Length-for-age and Weight-for-age percentiles

NAME _____

RECORD # _____

Revised April 20, 2001.
SOURCE: Developed by the National Center for Health Statistics in collaboration with
the National Center for Chronic Disease Prevention and Health Promotion (2000).
http://www.cdc.gov/growthcharts

CDC

Boys: Birth to 36 Months

High-fiber cereals,

Birth to 36 months: Boys
Length-for-age and Weight-for-age percentiles

NAME _____

RECORD # _____

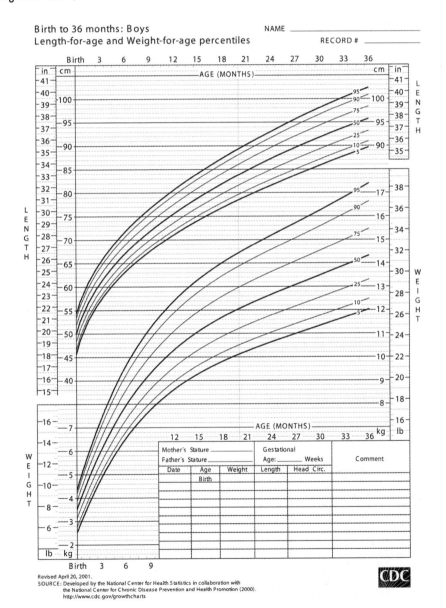

CDC

Girls 2 to 20 years:
Stature and weight for age

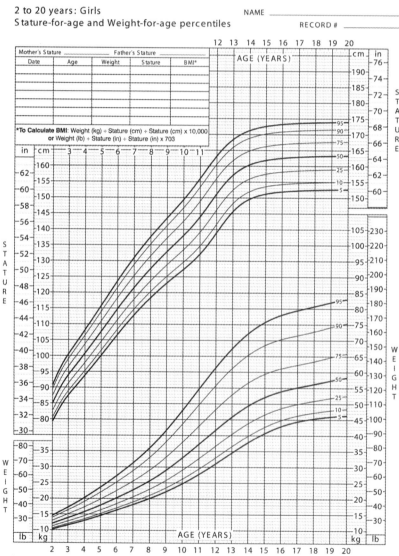

2 to 20 years: Girls
Stature-for-age and Weight-for-age percentiles

NAME

RECORD #

*To Calculate BMI: Weight (kg) ÷ Stature (cm) ÷ Stature (cm) x 10,000
or Weight (lb) ÷ Stature (in) ÷ Stature (in) x 703

Revised and corrected November 21, 2000.

SOURCE: Developed by the National Center for Health Statistics in collaboration with
the National Center for Chronic Disease Prevention and Health Promotion (2000).
http://www.cdc.gov/growthcharts

Girls 2 to 20 years: BMI Chart

2 to 20 years: Girls
Body mass index-for-age percentiles

NAME _____

RECORD # _____

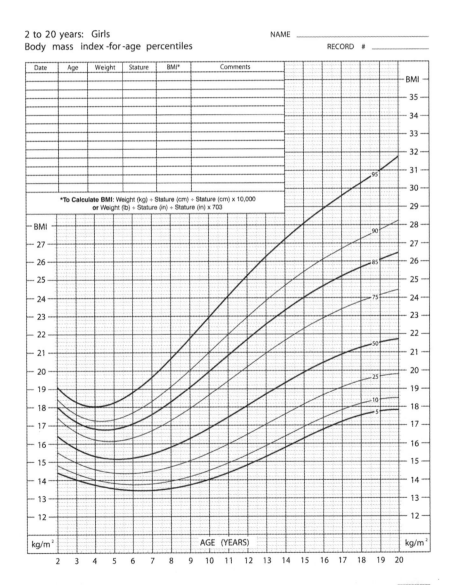

*To Calculate BMI: Weight (kg) ÷ Stature (cm) ÷ Stature (cm) x 10,000
or Weight (lb) ÷ Stature (in) ÷ Stature (in) x 703

SOURCE: Developed by the National Center for Health Statistics in collaboration with the National Center for Chronic Disease Prevention and Health Promotion (2000).
http://www.cdc.gov/growthcharts

Boys 2 to 20 years: Stature and weight for age

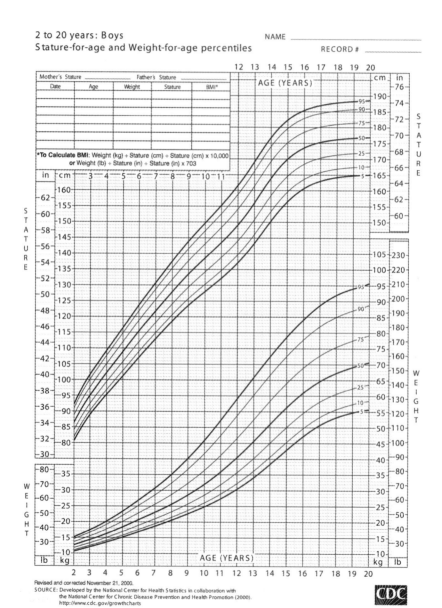

2 to 20 years: Boys
Stature-for-age and Weight-for-age percentiles

NAME _____

RECORD # _____

*To Calculate BMI: Weight (kg) ÷ Stature (cm) ÷ Stature (cm) x 10,000
or Weight (lb) ÷ Stature (in) ÷ Stature (in) x 703

Revised and corrected November 21, 2000.
SOURCE: Developed by the National Center for Health Statistics in collaboration with
the National Center for Chronic Disease Prevention and Health Promotion (2000).
http://www.cdc.gov/growthcharts

Boys 2 to 20 years: BMI Chart

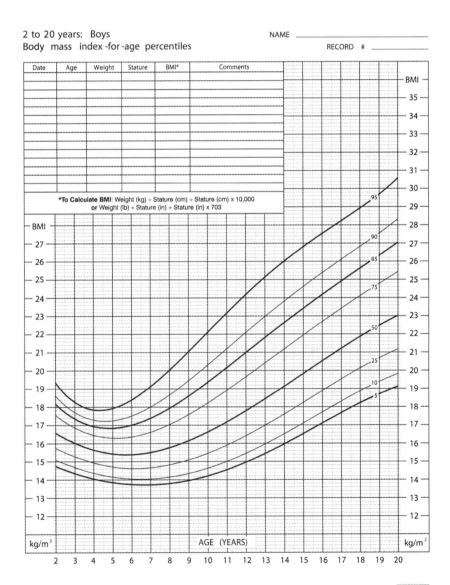

2 to 20 years: Boys
Body mass index-for-age percentiles

NAME _____

RECORD # _____

*To Calculate BMI: Weight (kg) ÷ Stature (cm) ÷ Stature (cm) x 10,000
or Weight (lb) ÷ Stature (in) ÷ Stature (in) x 703

AGE (YEARS)

SOURCE: Developed by the National Center for Health Statistics in collaboration with the National Center for Chronic Disease Prevention and Health Promotion (2000). http://www.cdc.gov/growthcharts

APPENDIX

 High Fiber
Foods

Food Source	Serving Size	Grams of Dietary Fiber
High-fiber cereals, like All-Bran	1/2 cup	10-14
Barley	1/2 cup	8
Wheat bran	1/2 cup	7
Kidney beans	1/2 cup	7
Chickpeas (garbanzo)	1/2 cup	7
Almonds roasted	2 oz. dry roasted 7	7Peanuts 2 oz. dry
Lima beans	1/2 cup	6
Navy beans	1/2 cup	6
Whole wheat pita bread	1 piece	5
Corn	1 ear	5
Carrot	1 medium, raw	3
Apple	1 medium	3
Banana	1 large	3
Kiwi	1 large	3
Pear	1 medium	3
Potato with skin	1 medium	2.5
Broccoli	1/2 cup	2
Popcorn	2 cups popped	2
Strawberries	1/2 cup	2
Apricots	5 dried halves	1.5

Source: Journal of the American Dietetic Association, June 1986 and October 1995
RDA for fiber is 25 grams for adults
Fiber requirements for children=child's age in years + 5

APPENDIX

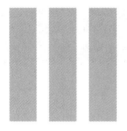

Calcium Requirements and Calcium Rich Foods

Calcium Dietary Reference Intake (DRI)

Age	*AI (mg/day)
0 to 6 months	210
6 to 12 months	270
1 to 3 years	500
4 to 8 years	800
9 to 18 years	1,300
19 to 50 years	1,000
51+ years	1,200

* Adequate Intake
Note that these apply to males and females. Lactating and pregnant women should consume the levels appropriate for their age.

Calcium Foods

Calcium Rich Foods	Amount	Mg Calcium
Broccoli, fresh, cooked	1/2 cup	89
Cheddar cheese	1 oz	205
Collards, fresh, cooked	1/2 cup	179
Milk, 1%	1 cup	300
Milk, 2%	1 cup	352
Milk, skim	1 cup	316
Mozzarella cheese	1 oz	207
Salmon, canned	3 oz	191
Sardines, canned	3 oz	372
Swiss cheese	1 oz	220
Tofu	1/2 cup	118
Yogurt, plain, low-fat	4 oz	207

APPENDIX IV

Food Guide Pyramid

A Guide to Daily Food Choices

Fats, Oils, & Sweets
Use Sparingly

KEY
■ **Fat** (naturally occuring and added)
▼ **Sugars** (added)
These symbols show that fat and added sugars come mostly from fats, oils, and sweets, but can be part of or added to foods from the other food groups as well.

Milk, Yogurt,
& Cheese Group
2–3 Servings

Meat, Poultry, Fish,
Dry Beans, Eggs,
& Nuts Group
2–3 Servings

Vegetable
Group
3–5 Servings

Fruit Group **2–4**
Servings

Bread, Cereal,
Rice, & Pasta
Group
6–11
Servings

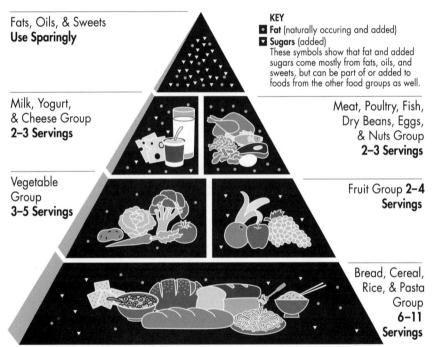

SOURCE: U.S. Department of Agriculture/U.S. Department of Health and Human Services

Kids Eat Great and Love It!

APPENDIX

V

Breastfeeding Resources

La Leche League International

1400 North Meacham Road
Schaumburg, IL 60173-4840

> Referral to local support groups:
> (800) LA LECHE
>
> General information:
> (847) 518-7730
>
> Recorded information on selected breastfeeding topics:
> (900) 448-7475 ext. 27

To locate a lactation consultant:

> International Lactation Consultant Association
> (312) 541-1710
>
> Medela, Inc.
> (800) TELL YOU

Professional advice on breastfeeding:

> Center for Breastfeeding Information
> (847) 519-7730 ext. 245 or 241

Information on medications and breastfeeding:

> Rocky Mountain Drug Consultation Center
> (900) 370-3784

Web sites with breastfeeding information:

> www.bflrc.com
>
> Bright Future Lactation Resource Centre. Supportive education and motivation for those who are breastfeeding.
>
> www.breastfeeding.com
>
> Support for all aspects of breastfeeding.

APPENDIX VI

Organic Foods and Nutritional Products

Organic Foods

If organic foods are not readily available in your area try these companies. You may order on-line or order a catalog to place a phone order.

Garden Spot Distributors

438 White Oak Road
New Holland, PA 17557
Tel: (800) 829-5100 or (717) 354-4936
Web: www.gardenspotsfinest.com

An East Coast distributor that carries organic grains, breads, produce, dairy, poultry, and beef.

Jaffe Brothers, Inc.

P.O. Box 636
Valley Center, CA 92082-0636
Tel: (760) 749-1133
Web: www.organicfruitsandnuts.com

Offers organic greens, dried fruit, nuts, seeds, snack foods, grains, and pastas.

Nature's One

12 Westerville Square, Ste. 308
Westerville, OH 43081
Tel: (614) 898-9758
Web: www.naturesone.com

Offers organic, non-GMO baby formula as Baby's Only Organic brand. Dairy-based and soy available.

Organic Provisions

P.O. Box 756
Richboro, PA 18954-0756
Tel: (800) 490-0044 or (215) 674-2217
Web: www.orgfood.com

Offers a wide variety of organic and Kosher organic foods.

Village Organics

P.O. Box 4630
Davidson, NC 28036
Tel: (704) 504-2474 ext.205
Web: www.villageorganics.com

Offers a wide variety of organic foods.

Nutritional Products

These companies, through my personal research, follow high standards for quality control of their products and screen raw ingredients for contamination.

Coromega

Tel: (877) 275-3725
Web: www.coromega.com

A fish oil supplement of DHA and EPA in an orange-flavored, pudding-like emulsion. Mix with yogurt or smoothies for children.

Martek BioSciences Corporation

Tel: (410) 740-0081
Web: www.martekbio.com

The manufacturer of DHA and AA oils added to infant formulas around the world. Also has a chewable DHA supplement, called *Neuromins DHA*.

Triceram Cream

Tel: (800) 440-1441
Web: www.osmotics.com

A non-steriodal, natural lipid moisturizer that aids in healing eczema.

USANA Health Sciences

Tel: (888) 953-9595
Web: www.usana.com

Vitamin-mineral supplements for children, teens, and adults. Children's chewable vitamins sweetened with xylitol (see p. 162). Fish oil products screened for contamination. Excellent grape seed extract combined with vitamin C.

APPENDIX VII

Suggested Reading and Web Sites

Books

Bionutrition: Winning the War Within

Ray Strand, M.D.
Comprehensive Wellness Publishing, 1998
Call (800) 723-8446 to order

Delves into the role of nutritional supplementation for adults and how this impacts disease.

Down to Earth

Michael J. Rosen
Harcourt Brace, 1998
Ages 6 and up

Contains gardening stories and projects for kids.

The Glucose Revolution

Jennie Brand-Miller Ph.D., Thomas M.S. Wolever, M.D., Ph.D.
Marlowe and Company, 1999

A comprehensive book about the glycemic index and how controlling blood sugar can help with weight loss, improve athletic performance, and manage diabetes.

Healthy School Lunch Action Guide

Susan Campbell and Todd Winant
Earth Save Foundation, 1994
Call (408) 423-4069 to order

Information to guide parents in making changes in their school lunch program.

The Healthy Start Kids' Cookbook

Sandra K. Nissenberg
Chronimed, 1994

Fun, tasty, and healthy recipes kids can make themselves.

How to Get Your Kid to Eat ... But Not Too Much

Ellyn Satter
Bull Publishing, 1987

A guide for feeding children of all ages.

Is This Your Child?

Doris Rapp, M.D.
William Morrow and Company, 1992

How to recognize food and environmental factors that can affect behavior.

KidShapes

Laura Walther Nathanson, M.D.
Harper Collins, 1995

A guide to childhood weight control.

Super Baby Food

Ruth Yaron
F. J. Publishing Company, 1998

Everything you need to know about making homemade baby foods.

Vegetables Rock – A Guide for Teenage Vegetarians

Stephanie Pierson
Bantam, 1998

Advantages of eating right as a vegetarian with information on basic nutrition, junk food, fast food, and health food for teens.

Web Sites

CDC Growth Charts

www.cdc.gov/growthcharts/

Access to height, weight, and body mass index growth charts for children.

The Center for Eating Disorders

www.eating-disorders.com

Find information about eating disorders and join a discussion group.

Call Your Pediatrician

www.callyourped.com

Information on common childhood illnesses, written by Dr. Wood.

Center for Science in the Public Interest

www.cspinet.org

A nonprofit organization that researches safety and nutritional quality of the food supply.

Children and Adults with Attention-Deficit/Hyperactivity Disorder

www.chadd.org

(800) 233-4050

Information on finding a local support group for families dealing with ADD.

Consumers Union

www.consunion.org

Information from the group that publishes Consumer Reports. Their report, "Do You Know What You're Eating? An Analysis of US Government Data on Pesticide Residues in Foods" is available on-line.

Environmental Working Group

www.ewg.org

Web site with information about environmental awareness.

Kids Eat Great

www.kidseatgreat.com

Dr. Wood's site with excerpts from this book, her schedule of events, and information about her nutritional program for overweight children. Sign up for a free nutritional newsletter.

National Association of Anorexia Nervosa and Associated Disorders

www.anad.org

(847) 831-3438

Contact to receive a listing of support groups and referrals for eating disorders.

Something Fishy

www.something-fishy.org

A site all about eating disorders.

Weight-Control Information Network (WIN)

www.niddk.nih.gov/health/nutrit/win.htm

(301) 984-7378 or (800) 946-8098

E-mail: win@info.niddk.nih.gov

Help with finding a pediatric weight-control program.

references
General References

Carper, Jean. *Miracle Cures.* New York: HarperCollins Publisher, 1998.

Carper, Jean. *Total Nutrition Guide.* New York: Bantam Books, 1987.

Consumer Reports. Organic Food: Greener greens? Volume 63, no. 1, January 1998. p. 12-18.

Consumer Reports. How Safe is Our Produce? Volume 64, no. 3, March 1999. p. 28-31.

Cooper, Kenneth. *Advanced Nutritional Therapies.* Nashville, Tenn: Thomas Nelson, Inc., 1996.

Galland, Leo. *Superimmunity for Kids.* New York: Copestone Press, Inc., 1988.

Mindell, Earl L. *Parents' Nutrition Bible.* Carlsbad, Ca: Hay House, Inc., 1992.

Nathanson, Laura. *No More Babyfat!* New York: Harper Perrenial, 1995.

Passwater, Richard A. *Fish Oil Update.* New Canaan, Conn: Keats Publishing, 1987.

Satter, Ellyn. *How to Get Your Kid to Eat . . . But Not Too Much.* Palo Alto, Ca: Bull Publishing, 1987.

Steinberg, Laurence and Ann Levine. *You and Your Adolescent.* New York: Harper Perrenial, 1987.

Strand, Ray. *Bionutrition:Winning the War Within.* Rapid City, SD: Comprehensive Wellness Publishing, 1998.

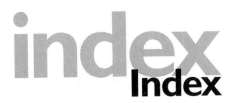

Index

footnotes
Footnotes

Chapter 1

1.Mu~noz KA, Krebs-Smith SM et al. Food intakes of US children and adolescents compared with recommendations. *Pediatrics.* 1997;100:323-329.

2.Dietz WH. Health consequences of obesity in youth: predictors of adult disease. *Pediatrics.* 1998;101S(3):518S-525S.

3.*The Surgeon General's Report on Nutrition and Health.* Public Health Service, US Department of Health and Human Services. 1988;2.

4.Miller, BA et al. SEER Cancer Statistics Review 1973-1990. NIH. 1993; pub. no. 93-2789.

5.Harel Z, Riggs S et al. Adolescents and calcium: what they do and do not know and how much they consume. *J Adolesc Health.* 1998;22(3):225.

6.Hill JO and Trowbridge FL. Childhood obesity: Future directions and research priorities. *Pediatrics.* 1998;101S:570-574.

7.Rosenbaum M, Rudolph LL. The physiology of body weight regulation: relevance to the etiology of obesity in children. *Pediatrics.* 1998;101S:525-539.

8.Ross JG, Dotson CO, Gilbert GG, Katz SJ. What are kids doing in school physical education? *J Phys Ed Recr Dance.* 1985;56:35-39.

9.Dietz WH, Gortmaker SL. Do we fatten our children at the television set? Obesity and television viewing in children and adolescents. *Pediatrics.* 1985; 75:807-812.

10.Townsend MS, Peerson J et al. Food insecurity is positively related to overweight in women. *J. Nutr.* 2001;131:1738-1745.

11.McGinnis JM, Foege WH. Actual causes of death in the United States. *JAMA.* 1993;280:2207-2211.

12.Carmargo C. American Lung Association/American Thoracic Society International Conference. April 1999.

13.Manson JE, Willett WC, Stampfer MJ et al. Body weight and mortality among women. *N Engl J Med.* 1995;333:677-85.

14.Must AV et al. Long term morbidity and morbidity of overweight adolescents. *N Engl J Med.* 1992;327:1350.

15.Report from the Center for Science in the Public Interest (CSPI). October 22, 1998.

16.Dennison BA, Rockwell HL, Baker SL. Fruit and vegetable intake in young children. *J Am Coll Nutr.* 1998;17:371-378.

17.Krebs-Smith SM, A Cook et al. Fruit and vegetable intakes of children and adolescents in the United States. *Arch Pediatr Adolesc Med.* 1996;150:81-86.

18.Subar AF, Krebs-Smith SM et al. Dietary sources of nutrients among US children: 1989-1991. *Pediatrics.* 1998;102:913-923.

19.Strong JP, Malcom GT et al. Early lesions of atherosclerosis in childhood and youth: natural history and risk factors. *J Am Coll Nutr.* 1992;11S:51S-54S.

20.Strong JP, Malcom GT et al. Prevalence and extent of atherosclerosis in adolescents and young adults: implications for prevention from the pathobiological determinants of atherosclerosis in youth study. *JAMA.* 1999;281:727-735.

21.Gillman MW, Cupples LA et al. Protective effect of fruits and vegetables on development of stroke in men. *JAMA.* 1995;273:1113-1117.

22.Ames BN. Ames agrees with mom's advice: eat your fruits and vegetables. *JAMA.* 1995;273:1077-1078.

Chapter 2

23.www.consunion.org. February 7, 1999.

24.Nowhere to Hide: Persistent Toxic chemicals in the U.S. food Supply. *Pesticide Action Network North America.* March 2001. www.panna.org

25.www.ewg.org. February 7, 1999.

26.Leiss JK, Savitz DA. Home pesticide use and childhood cancer: a case-control study. *Am J Public Health.* 1995; 85:249-252.

27.Daniels JL, Olshan AF, Savitz DA. Pesticides and childhood cancers. *Environ Health Perspect.* 1997;105:1068-1077.

28.Longnecker MP, Rogan WJ and Lucier G. The human health effects of DDT and PCBs and an overview of organochlorines in public health. *Annu Rev Public Health.* 1997;18:211.

29. Buck GM, Vena J et al. Parental consumption of contaminated sport fish from Lake Ontario and predicted fecundability. *Epidemiology.* 2000;11:388-393.

30.www2.nas.edu/whatsnew/28ea.html. March 14, 1999.

31.Willet WC, Stampfer MJ et al. Relationship of meat , fat, and fiber intake in the risk of colon cancer in a prospective study among women. *N Engl J Med.* 1990;323:1664-1772.

32.Bernard S, Enayati, A et al. Autism: a Novel Form of Mercury Poisoning. July 2000. http://www.autism.com/ari/mercury.html

33.US Geological Survey, *The quality of our nation's waters (1999).* http:/water.usgs.gov/pubs/circ/circ1225/. March 14, 1999.

34.www.ewg.org. February 7, 1999.

Chapter 3

35.Hornick S. Factors affecting the nutritional quality of crops. *Am J Altern Agriculture.* 1992;7:1.

36.Oakley GP. Eat right *and* take a multivitamin. *N Engl J Med.* 1998;338:1060-1061.

37.Chandra RK. Graying of the immune system: can nutrient supplements improve immunity in the elderly? *JAMA.* 1997;277:1398-1399.

38.Mehta J. Intake of antioxidants among American cardiologists. *Am J Cardiol.* 1997;79:1558-1560.

39.Slesinski MJ, Subar AF, Kahle LL. Dietary intake of fat, fiber and other nutrients is related to the use of vitamin and mineral supplements in the United States: The 1992 National Health Interview Survey. *J Nutr.* 1996;126:3001-3008.

40.Abbott RD, White LR et al. Height as a marker of childhood development and late-life cognitive function: the Honolulu-Asia Aging Study. *Pediatrics.* 1998;102:602-609.

41.Sazawal S, Black RE et al. Zinc supplementation reduces the incidence of acute lower respiratory infections in infants and preschool children. *Pediatrics.* 1998;102:1-5.

42.Blusztajn JK. Choline, a vital amine. *Science.* 1998;281:794-795.

43.Heilman JR, Kiritsy MC et al. Fluoride concentrations of infant foods. *J Am Dent Assoc.* 1997;128:857-863.

44.Walter T, Dallman PR, Pizarro F et al. Effectiveness of iron-fortified infant cereal in prevention of iron deficiency anemia. *Pediatrics.* 1993;91:976-982.

45.Renaud S, Paul T. Cretan Mediterranean diet for prevention of coronary heart disease. *Am J Clin Nutr.* 1995;61(suppl):1360S-1367S.

46.Birch DG, Borch EE et al. Retinal development in very-low-birth-weight infants fed diets differing in omega-3 fatty acids. *Invest Opthalmol Vis Sci.* 1992;33:2365-2376.

47.Makrides M, Neumann MA, Gibson RA. Are long-chain polyunsaturated fatty acids essential nutrients in infancy? *Lancet.* 1995;345:1463-1468.

48.Willatts P, Forsyth JS et al. Effect of long-chain polyunsaturated fatty acids in infant formula on problem solving at 10 months of age. Lancet. 1998;352:688-691.

49.Pisacane A, Impagliazzo N et al. Breast feeding and multiple sclerosis. *BMJ.* 1994;308:1411-1412.

Chapter 4

50.Horwood LJ, Fergusson DM. Breastfeeding and later cognitive and academic outcomes. *Pediatrics.* 1998;101:99-100.

51.Kajosaari M, Saarinen U et al. Prophylaxis of atopic disease by six months' total solid food elimination. Evaluation of 135 exclusively breastfed infants of atopic families. *Acta Paediatr Scand.* 1983;72:411-414.

52.Halken S, Host A, Hansen LG, et al. Effect of an allergy prevention program on incidence of atopic symptoms in infancy. *Ann Allergy.* 1992;47:545-553.

53.Saarinen UM, Kajosaari M. Breastfeeding as prophylaxis against atopic disease: prospective follow-up until 17 years old. *Lancet.* 1995;346:1065-1069.

54.Lawrence, Ruth A. *Breastfeeding: A Guide for the Medical Profession.* St. Louis:C.V.Mosby, 1989. p. 246.

55.Dewey K and McCrory M. Effects of dieting and physical activity on pregnancy and lactation. *Am J Clin Nutr.* 1994;59(Suppl):446S-459S.

Chapter 5

56.Fomon SJ. *Nutrition of Normal Infants.* St. Louis, MO:Mosby-Year Book 1993. p.443-454.

57.www.ewg.org/pub/home/Reports/Baby_Food/Baby_Home.html. August 15, 2001.

Chapter 8

58.Rask-Nissila L, Jokinen E et al. Neurological development of 5-year-old children receiving a low-saturated fat, low-cholesterol diet since infancy. *JAMA.* 2000;284:993-1000.

59.Birch LL, Marlin DW. I don't like it; I never tried it: effects of exposure to food on two-year-old children's food preferences. *Appetite.* 1982;4:353-360.

60.Hammer LD, Bryson S, Agras WS. Development of feeding practices during the first five years of life. *Arch Pediatr Adol Med.* 1999;153:189-194.

61.Johnson SL, McPhee L, Virch LL. Conditioned preferences: young children prefer flavors associated with high dietary fat. *Physiol Behav.* 1991;50:1245-1251.

Chapter 9

62.Guo SS, Roche AF et al. The predictive value of childhood body mass index values for overweight at age 35 y. *Am J Clin Nutr.* 1994;59:810-819.

63.Cotugna N. TV ads on Saturday morning children's programming: what's new? *J Nutr Educ.* 1988;20:125-127.

64.Birch LL. Effects of peer models' food choices and eating behaviors on preschoolers' food preferences. *Child Dev.* 1980;51:489-496.

Chapter 10

65.Dennison BA, Rockwell HL, Baker SL. Fruit and vegetable intake in young children. *J Am Coll Nutr.* 1998;17:371-378.

66.Sinaiko AR, Donahue RP et al. Relation of increase in weight during childhood and adolescence to body size, blood pressure, fasting insulin and lipids in young adults. *Circulation.* 1999;99:1471-1476.

67.Kinter M, Boss PG, Johnson N. The relationship between dysfunctional family environments and family member food intake. *J Marriage and Family.* 1981;43:633-641.

68.Dwyer JT, Stone EJ et al. Predictors of overweight and overfatness in a multiethnic pediatric population. Child and Adolescent Trial for Cardiovascular Health Collaborative Research Group. *Am J Clin Nutr.* 1998;67:602-610.

Chapter 11

69.Feunekes GI, de Graaf C et al. Food choice and fat intake of adolescents and adults: associations of intakes within social networks. *Prev Med.* 1998;27:645-656.

70.Harel Z, Riggs S et al. Adolescents and calcium: what they do and do not know and how much they consume. *J Adoles Health.* 1998;22(3):225-228.

71.Benton D and Parker PY. Breakfast, blood glucose, and cognition. *Am J Clin Nut.* 1998;67:772-778.

Chapter 12

72.Murata M. Secular trends in growth and changes in eating pattern of Japanese children. *Am J Clin Nut.* 2000;72(5 Suppl):1379S-1383S.

Chapter 13

73.Hatch GE. Asthma, inhaled oxidants, and dietary antioxidants. *Am J Clin Nutr.* 1995;61S:625S-630S.

74.Britton J, Pavord I et al. Dietary magnesium, lung function, wheezing, and airway hyperreactivity in a random adult population sample. *Lancet.* 1994;344:357-62.

75.Kadrabova J, Mad'aric A et al. Selenium status is decreased in patients with intrinsic asthma. *Biol Trace Elem Res.* 1996;52:241-248.

76.Cohen HA, Neuman I, Nahum H. Blocking effect of vitamin C in exercise-induced asthma. *Arch Pediatr Adolesc Med.* 1997;151:367-370.

77.Soutar A, Seaton A, Brown K. Bronchial reactivity and dietary antioxidants. *Thorax.* 1997;52:166-170.

78.Hodge L, Salome CM et al. Consumption of oily fish and childhood asthma. *Med J Aust.* 1996;164:137-140.

79.Trenga, Carol. American Lung Association/American Thoracic Society International Conference in San Diego. May 1997.

80.Middleton E, Drzewieki G. Flavonoid inhibition of human basophil histamine release stimulated by various agents. *Biochem Pharmacol.* 1984;33:3333-3338.

81.Hoppu U, Kalliomake M, Isolauri E. Maternal diet rich in saturated fat during breastfeeding is associated with atopic sensitization of the infant. *Eur J Clin Nutr.* 2000;54(9):702-705.

82.Horrobin DF. Essential fatty acid metablosim and its modification in atopic eczema. *Am J Clin Nut.* 2000;71(suppl):367S-372S.

Chapter 14

83.Yakinci C, Turgut M et al. Serum vitamin A and beta-carotene levels in children with recurrent acute respiratory infections and diarrhoea in Malatya. *J Trop Pediatr.* 1997;43(6):337-340.

84.Dudley L, Hussey G. et al. Vitamin A status, other risk factors and acute respiratory infection morbidity in children. *S Afr Med J.* 1997;87:65-70.

85.Sazawal S, Black RE et al. Effect of zinc on acute lower respiratory infections. *Pediatrics.* 1998;102:1-5.

86.Ruel MT, Rivera JA et al. Impact of zinc supplementation on morbidity from diarrhea and respiratory infections among rural Guatemalan children. *Pediatrics.* 1997;99:808-813.

87.Marshall S. Zinc gluconate and the common cold. Review of randomized controlled trials. *Can Fam Physician.* 1998;44:1037-1042.

88.Macknin ML, Piedmonte M et al. Zinc gluconate lozenges for treating the common cold in children: a randomized controlled trial. *JAMA.* 1998;279:1962-1967.

89.Hemil̈a H. Vitamin C and common cold incidence: a review of studies with subjects under heavy physical stress. *Int J Sports Med.* 1996;17:379-383.

90.Westerveld GJ, Dekker I et al. Antioxidant levels in the nasal mucosa of patients with chronic sinusitis and healthy controls. *Arch Otolaryngol Head Neck Surg.* 1997;123:201-204.

91.Uhari M, Kontiokari T, Niemeta M. A novel use of xylitol sugar in preventing acute otitis media. *Pediatrics.* 1998;102:879-884.

92.Beck MA, Nelson, HK et al. Selenium deficiency increases the pathology of an influenza virus infection. FAS*EB J.* 2001 15: 1481-1483.

93.Moore BC. Drug-Induced Nutrient Depletion Handbook, 1999-2000. 2000.

94.Hatakka K, Savilahti E et al. Effect of long term consumption of probiotic milk on infections in children attending day care centres. *BMJ.* 2001;322:1327.

Chapter 15

95.Safer DJ, Zito JM, Fine EM. Increased methylphenidate usage for attention deficit disorder in the 1990s. *Pediatrics.* 1996;98:1084-1088.

96.*Toxicol Industr Health.* 1998;34:85-101.

97.Guillette EA, Meza MM et al. An anthropological approach to the evaluation of preschool children exposed to pesticides in Mexico. *Environ Health Perspect.* 1998;106:347-53.

98.Albright CD, Tsai AY et al. Choline availability alters embryonic development of the hippocampus and septum in the rat. *Brain Res Dev Brain Res.* 1999;113:13-20.

99.Rowe KS. Synthetic food colourings and "hyperactivity": a double-blind crossover study. *Aust Paediatr J.* 1988;24:143-147.

100.Kaplan BJ, McNicol J et al. Dietary replacement in preschool-aged hyperactive boys. *Pediatrics.* 1989;83:7-17.

101.Wolraich ML, Wilson DB, White JW. The effect of sugar on behavior or cognition in children. *JAMA.* 1995;274:1617-1621.

102.Krummel DA, Seligson FH, Guthrie HA. Hyperactivity: is candy causal? *Crit Rev Food Sci Nutr.* 1996;36:31-47.

103.Boris M and Mandel FS. Foods and additives are common causes of the attention deficit hyperactive disorder in children. *Ann Aller.* 1994;72:462-468.

104.Carter CM, Urbanowicz C et al. Effects of a few food diet in attention deficit disorder. *Arch Dis Child.* 1993;69:564-568.

105.Egger J, Carter CM et al. Controlled trial of oligoantigenic treatment in the hyperkinetic syndrome. *Lancet.* 1985:1(8428):540-545.

106.Stevens LJ, Zentall SS et al. Essential fatty acid metabolism in boys with attention-deficit hyperactivity disorder. *Am J Clin Nutr.* 1995;62:761-768.

107.Bekaroglu, M et al. Relationships between serum free fatty acids and zinc, and attention deficit hyperactivity disorder. *J Child Psych and Psychia.* 1995;37:225-227.

108.Arnold LE. Megavitamins for MBD: a placebo-controlled study. *JAMA.* 1978;20:24.

109.Haslam RHA, Dalby JT, Rademaker AW. Effects of megavitamin therapy on children with attention deficit disorders. *Pediatrics.* 1984;74:103-111.

110.Sever Y, Ashkenazi A et al. Iron treatment in children with ADHD: a preliminary report. *Neuropsychobiology.* 1997;35:178-180.

111.Bruner AB, Joffe A et al. Randomized study of cognitive effects of iron supplemuentation in non-anemic iron-deficient girls. *Lancet.* 1996;347:992-996.

112.Toren P, Sofia E et al. Zinc deficiency in ADHD. *Biol Psychiatry.* 1996;40:1308-1310.

113.Kozielec T, Starograt-Hermelin B. Assessment of magnesium levels in children with ADHD. *Magnes Res.* 1997;10:143-148.

114.Carper, J. *Miracle Cures.* Harper-Collins Publishers. 1997. p.233-236.

Chapter 16

115.Strong JP, Malcolm GT et al. Prevalence and extent of atherosclerosis in adolescents and young adults. *JAMA.* 1999;281:727-735.

116.Osganian SD, Stampfer MJ et al. Distribution of and factors associated with serum homocysteine levels in children. *JAMA.* 1999;281:1189-1196.

117. Dwyer JT, Stone EJ et al. Predictors of overweight and overfatness in a multiethnic pediatric population. Child and Adolescent Trial for Cardiovascular Health Collaborative Research Group. *Am J Clin Nutr.* 1998;67:602-610.

118.Harrell JS, Gansky SA et al. School-based interventions improve heart health in children with multiple cardiovascular disease risk factors. *Pediatrics.* 1998;102:371-380.

119.Robinson K, Arheart K et al. Low circulating folate and vitamin B6 concentrations: risk factors for stroke, peripheral vascular disease, and coronary artery disease. *Circulation.* 1998;97:437-443.

120.Boushey CJ, Refsum H et al. Serum total homocysteine and coronary heart disease. *Int J Epidemiol.* 1995;24:1049-1057.

121.Stephens NG, Parsons A et al. Randomised controlled trial of vitamin E and patients with coronary disease: Cambridge Heart Antioxidant Study (CHAOS). *Lancet.* 1996;347:781-786.

122.Kugiyama K, Motoyama TJ et al. Vitamin C attenuates abnormal vasomotor reactivity in spasm coronary arteries in patients with coronary spastic angina. *Am Coll Cardiol.* 1998;31:980-986.

123.American College of Cardiology meeting New Orleans, March 1999.

124.Langsjoen PH, Folkers K. A six-year clinical study of therapy of cardiomyopathy with Coenzyme Q10. *Int J Tissue React.* 1990;12(3):169-171.

125.Davis D, Dinse GE, Hoel DG. Decreasing cardiovascular disease and increasing cancer among whites in the United States from 1973 through1987. *JAMA.* 1994;271:431-437.

126.Clark LC, Combs GF Jr, Turnbull BW et al. Effects of selenium supplementation for cancer prevention in patients with carcinoma of the skin: A randomized controlled trial. Nutritional Prevention of Cancer Study Group. *JAMA.* 1996;24:1957-1963.

127.Giovannucci E, Stampfer MJ et al. Multivitamin use, folate, and colon cancer in women in the Nurses' Health Study. *Ann Intern Med.* 1998;129:517-524.

128.Blot WJ, Li B et al. Nutrition intervention trials in Linxian China. *J Natl Cancer Inst.* 1993;85:1483-1492.

129.Zhang S, Hunter DJ et al. Dietary carotenoids and vitamins A, C, and E and risk of breast cancer. *J Natl Cancer Inst.* 1999;91:547-556.

130.Knekt P, Jarvinen R et al. Dietary flavonoids and the risk of lung cancer and other malignant neoplasms. *Am J Epidemiol.* 1997;146:223-230.

131.Shklar G, Schwartz J et al. The effectiveness of a mixture of beta-carotene, alpha-tocopherol, glutathione, and ascorbic acid for cancer prevention. *Nutr Cancer.* 1993;20:145-151.

132.Lockwood K, Moesgaard S et al. Apparent partial remission of breast cancer in 'high risk' patients supplemented with nutritional antioxidants, essential fatty acids and coenzyme Q10. *Mol Aspects Med.* 1994;15S:231S-240S.

133.Council for Responsible Nutrition. Optimal nutrition for good health:The benefits of nutritional supplements. www.crnusa.org. April 2, 1999.

NOTES

NOTES